DIY Baby!
Do It Yourself Baby!

DIY Baby!
Do It Yourself Baby!
Your Essential Pregnancy Handbook

Shelley S. Binkley, M.D.

iUniverse, Inc.
New York   Bloomington   Shanghai

DIY Baby! Do It Yourself Baby!
Your Essential Pregnancy Handbook

Copyright © 2008 by Shelley S. Binkley, M.D.

iUniverse books may be ordered through booksellers or by contacting:

iUniverse
1663 Liberty Drive
Bloomington, IN 47403
www.iuniverse.com
1-800-Authors (1-800-288-4677)

Because of the dynamic nature of the Internet, any Web addresses or links contained in this book may have changed since publication and may no longer be valid.

The information, ideas, and suggestions in this book are not intended as a substitute for professional medical advice. Before following any suggestions contained in this book, you should consult your personal physician. Neither the author nor the publisher shall be liable or responsible for any loss or damage allegedly arising as a consequence of your use or application of any information or suggestions in this book.

ISBN: 978-0-595-49851-2 (pbk)
ISBN: 978-0-595-61275-8 (ebk)

Printed in the United States of America

Acknowledgements

I could not have completed this book without the love, support, friendship, inspiration and hard work of Richard Baker, Debra Allred, Lesa Chesnut, Julie Gambino, Jeni Harvey, Lisa Treadway, Karen Knudsen, Dean McConnell, Gundunmar (Gummi) Sigurdarson, George Foster, and Vance Feast.

Thank you to Doug Ellis, Dharma Communications, for excellent photography.

I extend my deepest gratitude to all the lovely ladies who've allowed me the opportunity to participate in their births over the years. You have taught me life's greatest lessons …

For Grace and in loving memory of Ann.

Contents

"Nurture and honor your child and your spirit shines like the sun. It rebounds and ricochets like diamonds of light off snow. In your child you become bound for all time to the future of the universe …"

—Anonymous

"This book is perfect for those looking for pertinent information in a concise, yet entertaining vehicle. Dr. Binkley, who has seen pregnancy from both sides, comes at the subject from the standpoint that pregnancy is a natural process and not a 'condition' where providers are supporters and advisors, rather than meddlers."

—John C. Hobbins, M.D., Professor of Obstetrics and Gynecology, University of Colorado School of Medicine, Aurora, Colorado

"[DIY Baby!] was easy to read and understand, I did not feel too bogged down with "too much info". There are so many books that talk about being pregnant, but I have been disappointed with how many actually go into detail about fetal development and what is going on in your body … It is pretty amazing."

—Chandra Allred, Mom-To-Be (for the second time around)

As a nurse, I've been with Dr Binkley through the good and the bad experiences of pregnancy and child birth in the hospital for the past twelve years. Shelley has always provided highly skilled technical and compassionate care, focusing on the best possible outcome for mother and baby. She has captured her caring philosophy in this book, which is a *must-read* for those contemplating pregnancy and child birth.

—Jeni Harvey RN (working in Labor/Delivery, Post Partum and Normal Newborn)

Introduction

To the Reader

DIY Baby! is *your* pregnancy book. The content arose from questions you've asked me over the past fifteen years. I desire and welcome your additional questions and constructive input for future editions. I plan to release revised editions every one to two years as knowledge in the field advances and peoples' interests change.

A New Wellness Paradigm for Birth in the United States

Welcome to parenthood! My mission is for you to have a happy healthy pregnancy and a beautiful baby for you are about to embark on life's greatest satisfaction. This book is your road map to have the best pregnancy experience possible. While the twentieth century witnessed dramatic declines in maternal and infant mortality as a result of improved medical care, the twenty-first century presents novel challenges and opportunities. Some of these derive from within ourselves and we can exert complete control over them; while others arise from external forces. The three factors that will have the greatest impact on our health this century are lifestyle, finances, and technology.

I have delivered babies and cared for people for fifteen years and through the years I have learned we exert the greatest control over our health through our lifestyle. Here I define lifestyle as our work habits, eating habits, and exercise habits. Most illnesses are brought on by a chronically unhealthy lifestyle. It's those little decisions we make day-to-day that pile up over time and cause us to enjoy good health or suffer bad health: whether or not to work those two hours of overtime, what to choose for lunch from the cafeteria, whether or not to exercise that day.

Lifestyle

My desire to impart to you an insider's understanding of pregnancy and birth so you can take charge of your health engendered *DIY Baby! (Do It Yourself Baby!)*. Pregnancy is a physically stressed state for the body. It's a normal state, but it does test our physical limits which is why most pregnancy-related illness are a manifestation of or a first sign of common medical conditions such as diabetes, high blood pressure, and consequences of stress.

Over-eating causes diabetes and high blood pressure in the pregnant and non-pregnant state. It increases the risk of pre-eclampsia (high blood pressure), gestational diabetes, cesarean section, dysfunctional labor, infection, and heart disease. Over-work and stress cause preterm labor, high blood pressure, heart disease, anxiety, and depression, including post-partum depression. Inactivity exacerbates the ramifications of over-eating and over-work.

Finance

Finances may exert more impact on your health care decisions in the near future.

Health care expenditure occupies the largest portion of the gross domestic product. In itself there is nothing wrong with this as we are nothing without our health. More frequently our health care decisions are being determined by finances. Millions of people lack health insurance. Many people with insurance have "high deductible" plans and bear a greater percentage of the cost of medical care out of pocket. Many insurance plans exclude maternity and contraceptive coverage or require payment of extra premium to obtain such coverage.

The delivery of obstetric care is likely to undergo a major re-organization over the next ten years due to multiple pressures from various sources on the field of obstetrics. One possible scenario is the centralization of obstetric care in larger hospitals and the advent of "laborists" who just manage labor and do no prenatal care. Prenatal care may be assumed by obstetricians, family physicians, and certified nurse midwives who do not manage labor and delivery.

If labor and delivery care is assumed by laborists whom you've never met until you arrive at the hospital in labor, care may become less personal and more "institutionalized". Birth is a special and spiritual experience. It behooves you to have all the knowledge and confidence possible about the process to make it your own. *DIY Baby!* delivers.

Technology

Now is the best time in history to bear a baby in the developed world. Mortality rates of mothers and term infants are very low. The hospital "Maternity Ward" has evolved into the "Family Birth Place". The homey LDR (Labor, Delivery, and Recovery Room) has replaced the sterile "closet" tiled in puce where women labored on gurneys and were transported to an operating room to deliver strapped in stirrups with their legs in the air.

A paradigm shift has occurred in the mentalities of obstetric care providers and labor nurses. The paternalistic patient-doctor or patient-nurse model has been replaced and providers now view themselves as expert support personnel. They see their role as the imperative to create as safe, individualized and fulfilling a birth experience as possible for everyone who walks through their doors. Women and families are more empowered in their birth experience than they were fifty or even twenty years ago. They possess greater information about their options and are savvier.

We've spent enormous resources and training to make hospital delivery as much "like home" as possible with the safety net of proximity to emergency services. However, while some obstetric emergencies are indeed unpredictable, most are predictable based on easily identifiable risk factors. The truly dire emergencies such as cord accidents and massive placental separation have an incidence of slightly less than 1/1000 births and cannot be prevented and may not always be "rescued" by delivering in a hospital. Even if the baby is "physically" saved in such a situation, he may suffer irrecoverable mental damage and live out a short one-to-two year life in a vegetative state hooked up to machines.

Many obstetrical "emergencies" are actually "urgencies" which can be mitigated by changes in labor position or administering medication to stop labor and other conservative measures. Fetuses endure a great deal of stress during labor and they have an enormous capacity for recovery and regeneration. We've learned the brain is more capable of growth than we previously thought and we prevail intact not only because of but despite our efforts

Technology, which has been our greatest friend in the past century, is becoming one of our worst detractors. Ninety percent of the health care dollar is spent on the last six months of life; and a significant portion of the remaining ten percent is spent on permanently impaired premature babies. The 1996 cost of babies born between twenty-five to thirty-six weeks gestation rang up at $38,000,000. Present estimates put that figure at $2,000,000,000. We're spending enormous resources on the extremes of life.

Despite the technological advances made in medicine in general we have not been able to lower the U.S. preterm birth rate. It has remained about ten percent for the past fifty years and has climbed slightly during that period.

A phenomenon which I'll call the "medicalization" of life and death has seeped into our culture over the past century. In the past we used to die and were born in the home; we were cared for by relatives in the comfort and security of a familiar environment. Now we die and are born in hospitals. We are kept alive, often in a "vegetative" state at either end by machines connected to our bodies through tubes and wires. I ask is this the best way? How much value should we place on the quality versus quantity of life? When and how do we draw the line for a cost-benefit analysis? What other ways are there to be born and die? Is there a sweeter way?

Your Baby is Your Connection to the Future of the Universe

Life is ruled by passion, needs, and sometimes wisdom. The choice we make in bringing a child into the universe impacts everyone, most of all, the child whom we are creating.

DIY Baby!

Do It Yourself Baby! is not a missive for you to go out and have your baby in the back yard. It is intended to avail you of the tools to maximize your and your baby's health through the factors you can control and make the best of those you cannot control. I offer you a new wellness paradigm to approach your pregnancy in a proactive fashion. I empower you to assume responsibility for the health of yourself and your baby no matter where you plan to deliver. In DIY Baby I explore the option of home birth. Is it time to reconsider how we enter the world in this country? Can a select portion of the population safely deliver at home? Should they? What are the logistics? What are the selection criteria? What are the advantages and disadvantages?

Pregnancy can be a time of uncertainty and it doesn't help that all your friends and relatives feel compelled to divulge their worst horror story of their pregnancy, labor or delivery. Despite the availability of resources on the market my patients' questions have made me realize the existing materials do not convey the information in a manner that's readable or stays with you.

I hope this guide will give you, in a short time, a practical overview of what to expect from pregnancy and delivery. I wish to assuage your worries, as most of you will have normal vaginal deliveries. You will gain an obstetrician and mother's perspective and knowledge of pregnancy and birth.

If you're going to be a new dad, I hope to provide a guide to the changes in your wife's body, as well as a road map to how to navigate her hormonal and emotional changes; and your own changes in adapting to fatherhood.

For the scientifically curious I include some of the medical background on your symptoms.

I welcome your constructive input and questions for future editions of this book so feel free to contact me with comments. DIY Baby! is a new kind of pregnancy book intended to initiate a dialogue on one of life's greatest experiences, having a baby.

Above all this handbook will give you a sense of confidence and empowerment when it comes to your pregnancy and birth. I hope you enjoy the ride and happy new baby!

Chapter 1

The Case of the Missing Period

You've been trying for months only to be disappointed by the appearance of that red stain, but this time nothing's come when it was supposed to arrive and you think "at last!" Or perhaps you've been anxiously awaiting your period or dreading the lack thereof after that passionate night during which the covers ended up in a tangled mess on the floor as you and your partner threw caution out the window, hoping against hope … Either way, the stick is blue. Congratulations, you're pregnant!

At this moment you may be struggling with a number of mixed emotions; simultaneously excited and full of uncertainty. Creating a family is the culmination of many people's life's dreams and hopes. It offers unlimited promise to put our stamp on the world through forming and raising the people we think the planet needs. Bringing a child into the world can be life's biggest opportunity for a do-over: Right past wrongs, rectify mistakes; fix what you think your parents didn't get right for you. Yet while full of hope and anticipation it's fraught with anxiety and an unprecedented level of responsibility: Will our baby turn out all right? Will we have a boy or girl? Will I survive pregnancy/labor? Will my body (my wife's body) be ruined? How will it affect our relationship? *Will I be a good parent?*

Pregnancy is also a time of mystery. What's going on in there? How does a baby develop from essentially nothing? Can the baby hear us? What does the baby see, think, and feel? It's common to day dream about your perfect new baby—this book aims to help you have the healthiest and most worry-free pregnancy possible.

When am I due? Naegele's Rule

The first thing you'll want to know is "When is our baby due?" You can calculate your due date using **Naegele's Rule**. When was the first day of your last menstrual period? Figure your due date by adding seven days to the date and counting backward three months. For example, if your last menstrual period was

Naegele's Rule to determine due date:
- **First day of last menstrual period**
- **Plus seven days**
- **Minus three months**
- **That's your due date**

April 14, add seven days (the 21st) and count backward three months—March, February, and January. You're due January 21st. In the United states, pregnancy lasts a mean of 282 days (forty weeks) counting from the first day of the last menstrual period; or 266 days from fertilization. "Full term" is any pregnancy ending after thirty-seven completed weeks of gestation.

Keep in mind a "due date" is better thought of as a "due month". You can deliver anywhere from thirty-seven weeks onward. If you get to be forty-one weeks gestation and haven't yet delivered, your obstetric care provider will often talk to you about induction of labor—using medication to make it happen.

Obstetric care providers commonly use a pregnancy wheel to quickly figure due date and gestational age during your prenatal visits. These are inexpensive devices often manufactured by pharmaceutical companies. They are generally accurate, but can be off by as much as five days, depending on the clarity of printing and your ob provider's eyesight.

If you are uncertain about the first date of your last menstrual period, or if you have irregular menstrual periods, your obstetric care provider will usually use ultrasound to determine your gestational age and due date.

Early Ultrasound

Ultrasound done between six and twelve weeks gestation is used to measure the *crown-rump length*, or the distance from the top of the head to the bottom of the "rump". This measurement is accurate to within seven to ten days for the assessment of gestational age and expected date of delivery. Often

> *Implantation spotting* **can occur anywhere from six to fourteen days after fertilization and is often confused with a normal period.**

this ultrasound is done via the vagina: A special ultrasound probe is covered with gel and an ultrasound condom and inserted into the vagina to visualize the pregnancy, your uterus, and ovaries.

Using transvaginal ultrasound, an embryo can be reliably detected six weeks from the first day of the last menstrual period. A heart beat can be detected by ultrasound at seven weeks gestation; and an embryo with a head, spine, and paddle-shaped "limb buds" can be detected by eight weeks gestation. By twelve weeks gestation, one can see bony structures of the skull, spine, and limbs, as well as distinguish internal anatomy such as brain, heart, liver, stomach, and bladder.

In women with twenty-eight day menstrual cycles, ovulation occurs on day fourteen of the cycle. The egg is viable (able to be fertilized) for about twenty-four hours. Sperm, however, can live in the reproductive tract of a woman for up to six days. The most likely time to get pregnant is when intercourse occurs any time within the six days preceding ovulation. The time from ovulation to onset of menses is always a consistent fourteen days (luteal phase, latter half of the menstrual cycle). However, the time between onset of menstruation and ovulation is variable (follicular phase, first half of the menstrual cycle). Women with short menstrual cycles (i.e. twenty-four to twenty-six days) ovulate earlier in their cycle (i.e. on day ten to twelve) and can theoretically get pregnant if they have unprotected intercourse at the end of their menses.

All of the major organ systems and body parts develop in the first eight weeks following fertilization. This is the time at which embryos are most susceptible to toxic effects of external substances such as alcohol, recreational drugs, medications, and radiation.

What Causes Twins?

Twin pregnancies result from one of two processes: Two thirds of twins are *dizygotic* (non-identical): two eggs ovulate and each is fertilized by a sperm. *Monozygotic* twins (identical: one third of all twin gestations) occur after fertilization, when the egg begins to divide, usually at the two-cell stage. At this point, the blastomeres split and become two separate but identical blastocysts, going on to develop into two distinct embryos (see "Science Notes" for terms and details).

The most common cause of multiple gestations in the present time is in vitro fertilization and other assisted reproductive technologies to treat infertility.

Science Notes: What's going on in there?
From sperm and egg to embryo (see illustration next page)

Fertilization to Morula

Under normal circumstances only one sperm can fertilize one egg. The penetration of the egg by a sperm induces a process called the *zona reaction* which makes the egg unreceptive to other sperm. Fertilization usually occurs at the far end of the fallopian tube from the uterine cavity (the fimbria). The fertilized egg then travels the length of the fallopian tube and in the process divides into cells called *blastomeres* to eventually form a ball of cells called the *morula* (contains twelve to sixteen blastomeres).

Morula to Blastocyst

The first division to the two-cell stage occurs approximately thirty hours after fertilization; and the morula stage is reached at about seventy-two hours after fertilization. The cell walls of the morula become porous and coalesce so as to form a hollow ball of cells, the *blastocyst*, at about five days after fertilization.

Blastocyst to Embryonic Disc

One pole of the blastocyst contains a clump of cells called the *inner cell mass*—this will eventually become a flat pear shaped structure called the embryonic disc. The embryonic disc undergoes a number of cell division, folding of layers, and cell migrations to form the embryo. About six days after fertilization the blastocyst implants into the uterine lining. This is often accompanied by a small amount of bleeding that occurs at roughly the time one would expect onset of a menstrual period.

The developing embryo is swept along the fallopian tube by microscopic "fingers" called "cilia".

Blastocyst (@ 8 days)

Two cell stage (@ 30 hours after fertilization)

Morula (@ 4 days)

Fertilization

Fallopian Tube

Uterus

Myometrium (uterine muscle)

Endometrium (uterine lining)

Ovary

Implantation (@ 9 days)

Cervix

Fimbriae of Fallopian Tube (pick up ovulated egg)

Vagina

Fertilization to Implantation

Pregnancy Dating

Dating your pregnancy is the most important thing to establish in early pregnancy. It not only allows you to have an idea of when you'll deliver; it also allows your ob provider to assess and follow your gestational age throughout pregnancy. Gestational age is the duration of pregnancy and is referred to as _____ weeks and ____ days; for example "twenty weeks two days" or "20-2/7 weeks". Precise due dates and knowledge of gestational age come into play with complications of pregnancy such as preterm labor or the need to induce labor at term.

A number of criteria are used to establish your due date, the primary one being the first date of your last menstrual period. If you don't know this date or if you have very irregular periods, usually ultrasound will be performed to assist in assessing due date and gestational age. Ultrasound is more accurate for dating the earlier it is done. Before twelve weeks ultrasound is accurate to within seven to ten days; between twelve to twenty-three weeks, accuracy is ten to fourteen days; and twenty-four weeks and beyond, accuracy decreases to twenty-one days.

If your ultrasound dates vary by a number of days greater than the range of error for that time in gestation, your ob provider may revise your due date. For example, if your menstrual dates show you to be ten weeks along, but ultrasound reveals the presence of a seven week size embryo, your ob provider will

> **Accuracy of Ultrasound in determining gestational age/ due date:**
> **6-12 wks: 7-10 days**
> **13-22 wks: 10-14 days**
> **23-40 wks: 21 days**

probably use your ultrasound dates because they are three weeks off your menstrual dates.

However, if your menstrual dates put you at ten weeks gestation, and ultrasound reveals a nine week size embryo, your ob provider will likely keep your menstrual dates as the due date because the ultrasound date is within the margin of error for a first trimester scan (seven to ten days).

Folic Acid and Early Nutrition

Early in gestation the cells of the embryo are rapidly dividing, migrating, and growing into a formed fetus. The spine and nervous system are some of the earliest structures to develop—collectively they are called the *neural tube*. Folic acid is a B vitamin that is essential to cell division and growth. Inadequate folic acid can increase the risk of neural tube defects, in which the spinal tube fails to close properly, resulting in anomalies (birth defects) such as spina bifida (open spine) or anencephaly (absence of the brain). Neural tube defects are caused by a defective gene for the metabolism of folic acid; however, the presence of this gene can be overcome by folic acid supplementation.

Neural tube defects occur in about 1.4-2/1000 births. Women of normal weight should have a minimum of four hundred micrograms (mcg) or 0.4 milligrams (mg) of folic acid in their daily diet. This is the amount commonly found in women's multivitamins or prenatal vitamins. Green leafy vegetables, meats, and fortified cereals are common dietary sources of folic acid. It is important to have adequate intake of folic acid prior to conception an in early pregnancy because neural tube defects occur at approximately twenty-eight days after fertilization.

Increased weight can increase the risk of neural tube defects: if you weigh two hundred pounds or more, your risk of having a fetus with a neural tube defect increases by two-fold. You should be getting at least one milligram of folic acid in your daily diet. A prior history of a fetus with a neural tube defect increases the risk to three to four percent: If you've had a prior baby with a neural tube defect your daily folic acid intake should equal four milligrams.

Throughout pregnancy it is important to eat a common sense diet: well-balanced with lots of fruits and vegetables. Avoid fast foods, snack foods, and refined sugars.

Alcohol

It's not unusual to learn you're pregnant until weeks to months after a missed period. In the meantime you may have had a few drinks on social occasions. This will not doom you to having a child with fetal alcohol syndrome.

Fetal alcohol syndrome is thought to be caused by a consistent daily intake of alcohol (at least three drinks per day) throughout pregnancy or regular binge drinking (regular i.e. weekly intake of six or more drinks per occasion). Its most prominent features are decreased intelligence, behavioral problems, and abnormal facial structure. The exact mechanism by which alcohol causes this is not known, but it is thought to be dose-related. In other words the more consistent the alcohol intake, the higher the risk of fetal alcohol syndrome.

Tobacco

Smoking during pregnancy is associated with decreased fetal growth, preterm birth, and with SIDS (sudden infant death syndrome) in the early neonatal period. Quitting can be tough, but it's generally safer to use smoking cessation aids such as nicotine replacement or buporion (an anti-depressant) than it is to continue to expose yourself and your baby to all the toxins in cigarette smoke (carbon monoxide, toluene, plutonium and other carcinogens).

Drugs and Medications

Illicit drugs such as cocaine and methamphetamines can be very dangerous in pregnancy producing birth defects and extreme preterm birth. Prescription narcotics and sedatives can produce withdrawal syndromes in the newborn.

Many pharmaceuticals are safe in pregnancy. For example most over-the-counter cold remedies are innocuous. However, aspirin and ibuprofen should be avoided unless prescribed by your ob provider, as these can impact the amniotic fluid volume and the fetal circulation. Some prescription medications can cause birth defects so consult your ob provider about your prescriptions as soon as you are considering pregnancy.

How much weight should I gain?

The three life phases during which women gain weight are: adolescence, pregnancy and menopause. If you control your weight gain during pregnancy, you'll stave off the major culprit of "middle age creep" when those added pounds just seemed to have materialized out of nowhere by the time you hit forty.

Pregnancy weight gain occurs in fits and starts, rather than a smooth progression. You may find between some of your prenatal visits you only gain one or two pounds; at others eight. The majority of pregnancy weight gain occurs after twenty weeks. You may not gain much weight at all by twelve weeks gestation—or you may gain five to ten pounds during that time—either one is normal. The total weight you should gain depends in part on your starting weight or body mass index (BMI). Your body mass index is your weight in kilograms divided by your height in meters squared (kg/m^2). If you want to know your BMI to the decimal places, you can calculate it using the following formula:

Formula to Calculate Body Mass Index (BMI):

(Weight in pounds ÷ height in inches ÷ height in inches) × 703 = BMI.

Once you calculate your body mass index you can estimate how much weight you should gain in pregnancy.

Body Mass Index, Health Status, and Expected Pregnancy Weight Gain

Body Mass Index	Health Status	Pregnancy Weight Gain Should be ...
19-25	"Normal"	25 to 35 pounds
26-29	"Overweight"	15 to 25 pounds
Under 19	"Underweight"	28 to 40 pounds
Over 30	"Obese"	15 pound or less

What should you eat during pregnancy? For a good reference on what you should eat based on your age, height, pre-pregnancy weight, and activity level, go to the following website:

www.mypyramid.gov/mypyramidmoms

Composition of Maternal Weight Gain at Term

Composition of Pregnancy Weight	Weight at Term (pounds)
Fetus	7.5
Placenta	1.5
Amniotic Fluid	1.8
Uterus	2.25
Breasts	1
Blood	3.4
Extravascular Fluid (swelling)	3.5
Maternal Fat Stores	7.5
Total	@29

Exercise in Pregnancy

You can continue your pre-pregnancy exercise routine into pregnancy, with rare exceptions. However, you should maintain your heart rate at 140 beats

Exercise: Keep your heart rate at or under 140 beats/minute

per minute or below to prevent your skeletal muscles from "stealing" blood from the placenta. Short bursts above 140 beats per minute are probably inconsequential. However, avoid sustained exercise at this intensity. You can calculate your heart rate with a heart rate monitor, or simply count your pulse (found at your wrist or neck) for six seconds and multiply by ten to get your heart rate per minute.

Pregnancy is not the time to begin a vigorous exercise routine when your previous routine consisted of flipping the buttons on the remote from the vantage point of the couch. Exercise during pregnancy depends on your pre-pregnant conditioning. If you were a world-class tri-athlete prior to becoming pregnant, you can continue many of these activities at a moderate, but not competition level, throughout much of pregnancy. Consult with your practitioner on specifics.

However, if you become inspired by your new condition to take better care of yourself, and you resolve to start an exercise routine, the best exercise in pregnancy is walking. A good routine to work toward and sustain throughout pregnancy and postpartum is walking forty-five minutes five times per week. Walking keeps your heart rate in the aerobic (fat burning) range, and can keep you fit throughout pregnancy and lactation.

The most common excuse for not exercising is "I don't have the time." Just like anything else that's important, make the time. If you're a morning person, wake up an hour earlier. If not, walk on your lunch break or in the evenings after work. Research shows that morning exercisers are most consistent and have the best long-term success at sticking with a program. Walking is also great post-partum for staving off the baby blues.

Early Symptoms of Pregnancy: Zero to Six Weeks: Breast Tenderness, Missed Period, Genital Changes

Early in pregnancy you may feel no different and even wonder if you are pregnant. Many of the symptoms of early pregnancy are caused by rising levels of the pregnancy hormone,

> **Breast tenderness is one of the earliest symptoms of pregnancy.**

human chorionic gonadotropin or HCG. This hormone level is produced beginning with fertilization, then shoots up to peak at twelve weeks gestation. After twelve weeks HCG levels drop dramatically to a steady state by fourteen to sixteen weeks gestation, where they remain throughout pregnancy.

Breast Changes

The earliest signs of pregnancy are a missed period, breast tenderness, and genital changes. After fertilization, progesterone, another pregnancy hormone, rises and this produces breast tenderness, the onset of which occurs at about the time of the missed period. Breast tenderness is particularly noticeable at the nipple and areola; and is usually at its worst from the missed period through fourteen weeks gestation. At that point it subsides somewhat (but not to pre-pregnancy levels), only to increase again in the final month of pregnancy.

You do not need to do anything special to prepare your breasts for breast-feeding. Normal breast manipulation, i.e. with wearing a bra or during intercourse, will not produce any ill effects. However, excessive nipple and breast stimulation can produce uterine contractions, and late in pregnancy can even bring on labor. The best preparation for breastfeeding can really only be done after delivery by early lactation efforts and working with the baby to develop latch-on (the baby's suckling process). Do not purchase a nursing bra until after your milk has come in. This usually occurs three to five days after delivery. Purchasing a nursing bra before your milk comes in will usually result in an ill-fitting bra that is too small.

Breast size increases dramatically throughout pregnancy and when your milk comes in. Your lactation breast size cannot be predicted by your pre-pregnant breast size. Even small-breasted women can have large changes in breast size throughout pregnancy and lactation. Following weaning your breasts return to their pre-pregnancy size, although they may take on a slightly different shape.

Genital Changes

Aside from a missed period, you may notice a change in vaginal discharge. Some people experience no vaginal discharge to a white or mucusy discharge related to increasing progesterone and

> **Intercourse is safe during all stages of pregnancy.**

estrogen levels. Most people have some discharge that fluctuates throughout pregnancy.

You may also notice a short-term change in sex drive. This is often accompanied by engorgement of the vaginal tissues. The labia (vaginal lips) may turn a dusky rose color throughout pregnancy. The pregnancy hormones and anticipation of a new baby can temporarily increase sex drive.

Intercourse is safe during all stages of pregnancy unless you are experiencing complications of pregnancy and have been advised to refrain from intercourse by your obstetric care provider. There is no association between intercourse and miscarriage or preterm labor. However, it is not unusual to have cramping and/or spotting (dark brown, pink or a small amount of bright red) after intercourse in pregnancy. This is usually not cause for alarm but should be reported to your ob provider at your next prenatal visit. Mucusy discharge is also common after intercourse and should not be cause for alarm.

Cramping

Cramping is experienced frequently throughout pregnancy beginning with the missed period. You may feel "twinges" in the pelvis from the midline out to the hips, or even down the legs. This is due to the rapid growth of the uterine muscle and the stretching of the ligaments that support the uterus in the pelvis. Cramping is not cause for alarm unless it is accompanied by heavy, ongoing (lasting more than a few hours) bleeding resembling a period.

Early Symptoms of Pregnancy: Six to Fourteen weeks: Fatigue, Nausea, Spotting or Bleeding, Emotional Ups and Downs

Fatigue

It's no wonder you're tired! An entire formed fetus develops during the first three months of pregnancy from a mere sperm and egg. Although the baby gains the most weight during the last three months of pregnancy, the first three witness the most dramatic organ formation.

Fatigue usually begins between six to eight weeks, peaks at twelve weeks and subsides by fourteen and sixteen weeks. It roughly corresponds to the rise in the pregnancy hormone, HCG.

Don't be surprised if you get home from work every day and want to take a two hour nap. Indulge yourself. And don't use your weekends trying to catch up on all the house cleaning or activity you missed during the week. Listen to your body and if it tells you to sleep—sleep!

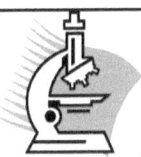

Science Notes: Behind the Fatigue: Embryo to Fetus

After implantation of the blastocyst, the inner cells mass evolves into the embryonic disc. This is a flat structure consisting of three layers of pluripotent (can form anything) embryonic stem cells: the ectoderm, mesoderm, and endoderm.

These stem cells undergo a miraculous process involving biochemical and bioelectrical cell-to-cell communication, cell migration, and differentiation (having a specific structure and function) to form all the major structures of a human being.

The ectoderm gives rise to the skin and nervous system; the mesoderm gives rise to muscles and bones; and endoderm gives rise to intestines, heart, and other internal organs. At nine weeks gestation the pregnancy transitions from the "embryonic" stage to the "fetal" stage.

It's no wonder you're fatigued as the embryo cells are multiplying by the thousands and hundreds of thousands per day. It takes a lot of energy to produce all these new cells. Even though the embryo is tiny, the magnitude of new cell production and growth is enormous.

Nausea

The onset and intensity of nausea also corresponds to the levels of the pregnancy hormone HCG. The term "morning sickness" is a misnomer—nausea can happen any time during the day. It's often brought on by not having eaten in two hours or more.

Nausea can be combated by eating small frequent meals—this seems to keep the stomach acids under control. If this fails wearing "sea bands" on your wrists (available at most pharmacies and supermarkets) makes use of an acupressure point for nausea. Nutritional supplements such as ginger and vitamin B6 help some women with nausea.

Consult your ob provider before taking over-the-counter or prescription anti-nausea medications. Many of these are safe but some are not.

Recalcitrant or unremitting vomiting resulting in an inability to tolerate liquids and solids needs to be addressed by your health care provider. If you have nausea to this degree your obstetric provider may prescribe an anti-emetic (medication to suppress nausea). Hyperemesis gravidarum is a rare condition of pregnancy in which nausea is so severe it involves recurrent hospitalization for intravenous fluids or nutrition.

Spotting and Bleeding

Most bleeding in early pregnancy does not signal a miscarriage. Twenty five percent of all women will have early pregnancy bleeding and go on to have uncomplicated normal term pregnan-

> **Most early pregnancy bleeding does not signify miscarriage.**

cies. Early pregnancy bleeding can range from a few days of spotting brown, pink, or red to what seems like a full blown period. This type of bleeding spans the range of normal. Often it is due to implantation spotting. Rarely, the rapid growth rate of the uterus versus the placenta can produce shearing forces that result in a small area of bleeding between the placenta and uterus called *subchorionic hemorrhage*. Subchorionic hemorrhage may be diagnosed on ultrasound by your ob provider. Most subchorionic hemorrhage heals without incident, and without resulting in miscarriage. However, if you are diagnosed with a subchorionic hemorrhage, you may be advised by your provider to refrain from intercourse until it has healed.

Consult your ob provider for bright red bleeding that lasts more than an hour and is accompanied by severe abdominal pain or intense cramping. These can signify a miscarriage or an ectopic pregnancy (pregnancy outside the uterus).

Emotions

Pregnancy throughout is accompanied by the full range of human emotions—sometimes vacillating from one extreme to another within minutes. The elation of the positive pregnancy test often gives way to anxiety about labor, pain; fear of the unknown, and concern about one's ability to be a good parent.

Don't be surprised if by eleven weeks gestation, when you're so tired it's all you can do to drag yourself out of bed, or you're so nauseous, you can't stand the thought of eating or not eating, you're asking yourself, "What have I done?" and "Can it be undone? I don't think I can go on with this." Ambiguity about pregnancy strikes late in the first trimester after the initial excitement has worn off and you realize you've got six to seven months more of this and then a new baby to deal with at the end of it all.

You may be wondering how your job or career will fit into your new family life. Who will stay home and take care of the baby? Will you send the baby to daycare or hire a nanny? If you have any concerns about you or your spouse's role in caring for the newborn, the earlier you initiate those discussions, the better. Some fathers will surprise you with their willingness to help out and their thoughtfulness to act without being asked. Others will disappoint in their lack of understanding and general cluelessness as to what needs to be done to most help you and the new baby. It may even be the same partner who exemplifies both!

Choosing your Ob Provider

There are many types of obstetrical care providers, each of whom has different training and areas of emphasis.

Obstetricians are M.D.'s or D.O.'s who've completed four years of medical school after college, followed by a four year residency in obstetrics and gynecology. They are highly trained specialists in women's health care and can handle normal pregnancy as well as any complication that may arise. They perform uncomplicated delivery as well as operative vaginal delivery (forceps and vacuum); and C-section when necessary.

Family physicians are M.D.'s or D.O.'s who've completed a family practice residency in addition to medical school. Some family practice residencies have a strong emphasis on obstetrics, while others do not, so their training is more variable. The obstetric focus in family practice training is normal uncomplicated pregnancy. Family physicians are not trained to do C-sections or operative vaginal deliveries, unless they complete additional training or a "fellowship" in obstetrics. Most family physicians have an arrangement with an obstetrician to cover complications that may necessitate interventions such as C-section or operative vaginal delivery.

Certified nurse midwives (CNM's) are advanced practice nurses who are registered nurses who have completed an additional two to three year program in nurse-midwifery. The focus of this training is normal pregnancy, although certified nurse midwives are trained in the complications of pregnancy and are competent to recognize and manage them. Certified nurse midwives are required to be licensed by the state, just as other health care providers such as physicians. Certified nurse midwives are often employed by physicians or hospitals to handle normal deliveries. They usually have a formal collaborative arrangement with an obstetrician to provide coverage for pregnancy complications or operative vaginal delivery/C-section if required.

Most obstetric care providers—obstetricians, family practitioners, and certified nurse midwives—work in groups to provide call coverage. You may be delivered by any one of the group members and you may not have a choice, depending on who's on call and how the group works its schedule.

In larger systems the prenatal care is often delivered by a mid-level provider such as a nurse practitioner or certified nurse midwife; and you may only see a physician in the latter part of pregnancy or in the hospital. If you choose to deliver at a teaching hospital you will likely be delivered by a resident (physician in training who has completed medical school). A medical student may also observe or attend your delivery. Junior residents are always "backed up" by senior residents and attending physicians so you will be well cared for should a complication arise.

Lay midwives and home births

Some people choose, for personal, religious, or financial reasons, to deliver at home with or without a birth attendant. Lay midwives or birth attendants may or may not have any formal training in obstetrics. Most women will deliver normally without complication and chances are, if you elect to deliver at home, you will have a healthy baby with no problems. However, the operative word there is "chance". If delivering at home, keep in mind a few things:

1) It will make a mess. Protect your bed or place of delivery with a water-proof sheet and be prepared to have a set of sheets/towels that will just need to be discarded afterward;

2) Monitor the baby's heart rate at least every five minutes during labor, and especially after each contraction. Many stores now sell hand-held "Doppler" fetal heart rate monitors. If the baby's heart rate drops repetitively during labor, you should proceed to the hospital for the health of your baby.

3) Emergency situations can arise quickly and without warning during labor; and you may or may not be able to get to the hospital in time to have a healthy baby and a healthy mom. This can include fetal intolerance of labor in which the baby does not get enough oxygen due to compression of the umbilical cord, separation of the placenta, or prolapse of the umbilical cord through the cervix. Severe bleeding may arise during and after labor, which may threaten the life and health of the mother and baby.

Obstructed labor in which the fetus gets "stuck" in the birth canal may cause fatigue to the baby; and may damage the maternal tissues such as the bladder. Prolonged pressure of the fetus on the mother's bladder or rectum may result in urinary or fecal incontinence (loss of control of urine or bowel movements) of the mother after delivery. This can be a persistent and severe problem to which the only solution may be surgery.

Modern obstetrical care whether delivered by a certified nurse midwife or physician has resulted in a maternal mortality rate close to zero. I recommend you avail you and your baby of this in one fashion or another. Prior to the 1920's the maternal mortality rate was as high as twenty-five percent; and the fetal/neonatal mortality rate was comparable.

Please read the chapters on labor and home birth before finalizing your decision to deliver at home.

Choosing where to deliver: Hospital or Birth Center

Most hospital obstetrics units now have "LDR's" which stands for Labor-Delivery-Recovery rooms in which you are admitted, labor, deliver, and recover all in one room. These are often decorated to have a "homey" atmosphere. Depending on the hospital you may have a limited or unlimited number of family members in the "LDR". The obstetrics unit usually has an operating room within the unit, or it is located close to the general operating suite, should you need a C-section.

Birth centers have similar LDR's, although they are not usually within the confines of a hospital. Birth centers will often be located adjacent to a hospital so you can be transported quickly to the operating room should the need arise.

In addition to your ob provider, your birth will be attended by one or more labor nurses. These are specialized nurses with training in labor and delivery, postpartum care, newborn care, and lactation. You will probably see more of your labor nurse during your stay, than you will of your midwife or physician. Your labor nurse is paid to attend you throughout your entire labor and to advise your ob care provider when his or her presence is necessary.

Your First Prenatal Visit

You've just missed your period, learned you're pregnant and you call your ob provider's office all excited only to be told, "Congratulations, we'll see you in six to eight weeks." They will

> **Your first prenatal visit is usually scheduled at ten to twelve weeks gestation.**

probably make sure you have a prescription for prenatal vitamins, give you miscarriage precautions and schedule you an appointment for when you're ten to twelve weeks gestation. Why don't they want to see you now? You certainly feel you must be seen right away as you've just learned you're pregnant! What could be more pressing or important?

Unless you've been struggling with infertility, had a history of recurrent miscarriage or a personal or family history of twins; or certain medical conditions such as high blood pressure, diabetes, or history of clotting disorders, your first prenatal visit is usually scheduled at ten to twelve weeks gestation. Why? That's when the first meaningful things can be learned about your pregnancy.

Wait a minute! Didn't I just spend a whole chapter telling you how all the crucial organ formation happens by twelve weeks gestation? Well, yes. But if something's going to go amiss with that process, there is really nothing you or your ob provider can do to prevent it from going awry. We can't give you medication or perform a surgical procedure to prevent a miscarriage, should one be in your future. Moreover, bed rest and pelvic rest (refraining from intercourse) have been proven to not prevent a miscarriage.

Ten to twelve weeks gestation is the first time the baby's heart beat can be discerned with a "Doppler". This is a device that amplifies sound and allows you and your ob provider to hear the baby's heart beat and confirm a living (viable) pregnancy. If you're going to have a miscarriage, it will usually occur before twelve weeks. It may or may not require special medical attention. However, if you're going to have a miscarriage after ten weeks, it likely will require medical intervention.

At the first prenatal visit, your ob provider will most likely do the following:
- A complete physical including a Pap smear and pelvic exam to confirm the size of your uterus is consistent with your pregnancy gestational age.
- Lab tests, including:

Blood type: You want to know if you're A, B, AB, or O in case you need a transfusion or if there's a rare problem after delivery called "ABO incompatibility".

Rh factor: You're either positive or negative for the Rh (Rhesus) factor. This is an antibody that you either make or don't make. If you don't make Rh antibody (are Rh negative) and you have a fetus who is Rh positive (has Rhesus protein on its blood cells) your antibodies to Rhesus factor can cross the placenta and lyse or "pop" the baby's blood cells, resulting in fetal anemia. If you are Rh negative, you will be given an injection called Rhogam at twenty-six to twenty-eight weeks gestation; or at any time in gestation if you experience significant vaginal bleeding; or if you have an amniocentesis. The purpose of the Rhogam injection is to prevent your body from developing antibodies to the Rh factor.

Blood Cell Antibodies: Included with your blood type, will be an "antibody screen". This evaluates your blood for rare antibodies that can react against proteins on fetal blood cells to cause anemia. This is similar to the test for Rhesus factor, but some antibodies can pose a greater threat to a developing fetus than Rhesus factor. These are extremely rare.

Hepatitis B Surface Antigen: You will be tested for hepatitis B because if you're positive for hepatitis B, the baby will be given hepatitis B immunoglobulin after birth. The helps protect the baby from contracting hepatitis during or following birth.

Syphilis screen (VDRL or RPR): It is important to screen for syphilis because it can be present without symptoms and it can cause severe birth defects. Asymptomatic syphilis is easily treated with antibiotics. If you have a positive VDRL or RPR the test will be confirmed with something called an "FTA-ABS". While former can have a high false positive rate (positive test with no disease), the latter is specific for detecting syphilis.

HIV test: The Centers for Disease Control (CDC) and the American College of Obstetrician-Gynecologists (ACOG) recommend universal screening of all pregnant women for HIV, regardless of risk factors. Don't be offended by your ob providers request to perform an HIV test. They are merely complying with the established national "standard of care". These national public health organizations recommend screening for HIV because treatment of HIV during pregnancy with anti-viral medications dramatically reduces the transmission of HIV from the mother to the fetus. The difference in transmission between treatment and non-treatment is so pronounced (from twenty-five percent to eight percent) that the initial study was terminated early because it was felt it was morally wrong to withhold treatment of HIV positive women after it was discovered that treatment produced such a profound reduction in the transmission rates from mother to baby.

Chlamydia/Gonorrhea: If you are between the ages eighteen and twenty-four, or have had multiple sexual partners, your ob provider may perform a culture for these sexually transmissible organisms. Some practices do this test on all pregnant women; others only do it for certain age groups or risk factors. It is not universally recommended by the CDC. These infections are easily treated with antibiotics. World-wide, Chlamydia is the number one cause of congenital (at birth) blindness.

Subsequent Prenatal Visits

You'll have on average, ten visits during your pregnancy if your first visit occurs between ten to twelve weeks. Between ten and twenty-six weeks, visits are monthly. From twenty-six to twenty-thirty six weeks visits occur every two weeks. After thirty-six weeks, visits are weekly.

After the initial set of labs, the other major labs are an ultrasound at twenty weeks (optional), gestational diabetes screening at twenty-six weeks, and screening for group B strep bacteria at roughly thirty-six weeks.

These labs may vary according to risk factors, age, and underlying medical illnesses.

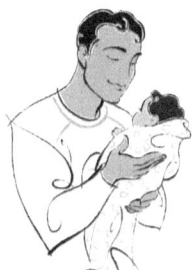

For Dads

For dads, even more so than moms, pregnancy doesn't seem real the first trimester. However there's a lot going on inside, despite lack of outer appearance of being pregnant. Mom may seem tired all the time, want to take naps and may not be interested in much. Her emotions may range from being excited about the pregnancy one moment to grumpy and irritable the next. The latter may be due to nausea, fatigue, or simple hormone fluctuations. On occasion, she may actually be more interested in sex than usual so make the most of the opportunity.

The best approach is to sit back, take things as they come, and not make too much of any one instant. Intensify the positive and minimize the negative.

Office Notes: Ambiguity about pregnancy; a common feeling

Kelsey is a thirty-five year old woman who had never been pregnant who came to see me. I had last seen her six months prior for depression.

"I think I might be pregnant but I can't remember when my last menstrual period was."

A urine pregnancy test confirmed it and ultrasound revealed she was six weeks along.

"I really don't want to be pregnant now. It's not the right time. I don't know how the baby's father is going to take it." She wasn't married to the father, in fact had been single all her life.

"I don't know how I feel about the baby's father. I mean I like him but…This may be my only chance at a baby, because I'm thirty-five you know."

Kelsey asked about options. I presented all the options to her in an informative, non-judgmental fashion.

As Kelsey left the office she said, "I just don't know what I'm going to do. I didn't plan on this but I may never have the opportunity again."

When women are feeling exhausted and sick, they often regret their choice to get pregnancy, even if it was a strongly desired pregnancy. This feeling usually passes by fourteen weeks gestation due to changes in hormones (see Chapter Three).

Kelsey showed up six weeks later for a first prenatal visit.

Chapter 2

Miscarriage and Early Pregnancy Loss Grief is Normal

Miscarriage is a common outcome of pregnancy. Having a miscarriage often triggers a lot of negative feelings like self doubt and guilt. However, there is almost nothing you can do to prevent it and it is a normal part of the spectrum of reproductive health. A miscarriage does not mean you'll never get pregnant again. Miscarriage is often nature's way of taking care of a pregnancy that wasn't developing properly.

Definitions

A miscarriage, also known as a *spontaneous abortion*, is a pregnancy that ends in embryonic or fetal demise before twenty weeks gestation with or without spontaneous expulsion of the pregnancy

> **Overall one in five pregnancies ends in miscarriage.**

tissue. A *complete abortion* is full expulsion of the pregnancy tissue. An *incomplete or partial abortion* is partial expulsion of the pregnancy tissue. A *missed abortion* is death of the embryo or fetus without expulsion of the pregnancy tissue.

Incidence and Causes

The risk of miscarriage increases with maternal and paternal age. It rises dramatically over age thirty-five. Twelve percent of pregnancies to women in their twenties end in miscarriage; this figure increases to twenty-six percent if over age thirty five. For paternal ages the rates are twelve percent and twenty percent respectively.

The increase in chromosomal problems with maternal and paternal age is due to "non-disjunction" or abnormal organization of the chromosomes (genetic material) during formation of the egg and sperm. An egg or sperm can end up with one too many, one too few, or an entire extra set of chromosomes.

More than half of all pregnancies ending in miscarriage are due to a major chromosomal abnormality. These include an extra chromosome (autosomal trisomy), a missing chromosome (monosomy—usually of the X chromosome), triploidy (three full sets of chromosomes), tetraploidy (four full sets of chromosome), and chromosomal "malformation" (structural abnormality of a chromosome).

Smoking increases the risk of miscarriage by twenty percent for each half pack a day inhaled. Consistent alcohol consumption of two drinks per week in the first eight weeks of pregnancy doubles the risk of miscarriage, and drinking daily triples the risk of miscarriage. The use of other drugs such as cocaine, amphetamines, and marijuana may increase the risk of miscarriage. These drugs, as well as tobacco and alcohol can cause later pregnancy complications.

Certain maternal diseases can increase the risk of miscarriage, most commonly insulin-dependent diabetes, and connective tissue disorders such as lupus. Hypothyroidism controlled with medication does not increase the risk of miscarriage.

The following activities do NOT increase the risk of miscarriage: drinking up to four cups of coffee or caffeine per day, sex, the rare alcoholic beverage, and maternal exercise. Maternal weight loss and weight gain in the first trimester are not associated with increased risk of miscarriage; however, maternal obesity (having a body mass index of thirty or greater) increases the risk of neural tube defects (improper closure of the spinal canal during development), which can in turn increase the risk of miscarriage.

Diagnosing Miscarriage

The symptoms of miscarriage are cramping (like intense menstrual cramps) and persistent vaginal bleeding like a heavy period. If you experience these in the first trimester, you should contact your practitioner. However, many people experience brief first trimester bleeding without having miscarriage, so most first trimester bleeding often does not signify impending miscarriage.

The typical course of a spontaneous miscarriage is to experience the onset of cramping and bleeding. Within a few hours the symptoms get very intense (like a mini-labor if you've already experienced labor). If the miscarriage completes spontaneously you may see passage of pregnancy tissue—it usually looks white or grey with clots. Subsequent to passage of tissue the bleeding and cramping subsides. Most spontaneous miscarriages take six to twelve hours to complete. You may still have bleeding like a light period for up to a week.

With an incomplete miscarriage you may have ongoing bleeding without passage of tissue. This should prompt you to contact your health care provider.

After a spontaneous miscarriage most people resume ovulation within three to four weeks. However, it is a good idea to wait through one or two normal cycles before attempting pregnancy again.

Treating Miscarriage

First trimester bleeding is so common it gives many people a scare. However, only twenty percent of people who experience first trimester bleeding will go on to have a pregnancy failure. Bed rest and pelvic rest (abstinence from intercourse) are often prescribed to prevent miscarriage in people who have first trimester bleeding but there is no evidence that these measures prevent an impending miscarriage.

Most miscarriages occur in the six to twelve week time frame and the entry point into the prenatal care system takes place at ten to twelve weeks gestation. Therefore, most miscarriages occur prior to seeing a practitioner for pregnancy care. So what do you do if you think you're having a miscarriage?

Spontaneous miscarriage does not need to be "treated". Most spontaneous miscarriages will complete without intervention. You should contact your health care provider if you are unsure you're having a miscarriage, if you think things are proceeding abnormally, or if you need reassurance about the miscarriage process.

> **Sex, exercise, and caffeine do NOT increase the risk of miscarriage.**

Some signs to be concerned about and prompt you to contact your health care provider are abdominal pain and/or ongoing cramping and bleeding lasting more than six hours without passage of tissue. These can signify an ectopic pregnancy or an incomplete miscarriage.

Ectopic Pregnancy

Abdominal pain can be a sign you have an ectopic or tubal pregnancy. Ectopic pregnancies are pregnancies not located in the uterus. The most frequent location for an ectopic pregnancy is in the fallopian tube. However, an ectopic pregnancy can be located anywhere, including the ovaries, the cervix, and the abdominal cavity. Ectopic pregnancies can be life threatening if they go undiagnosed long enough to rupture and cause internal bleeding.

If your practitioner suspects an ectopic or other abnormal first trimester pregnancy she may obtain an ultrasound and draw blood for a pregnancy hormone level to make the diagnosis. Ectopic pregnancy can be treated with medication if unruptured, but if ruptured or too large, needs surgical intervention.

Incomplete Miscarriage

An incomplete miscarriage often requires medical intervention, especially if you're having heavy bleeding.

Treatment of incomplete miscarriage varies depending on how much pregnancy tissue remains in the uterus. Retained pregnancy tissue can cause ongoing heavy bleeding so it is very important to remove all retained pregnancy tissue from the uterus.

If a minimal amount of pregnancy tissue remains in the uterus, sometimes misoprostol, or Cytotec, a drug used for labor induction, is used to encourage the uterus to expel the remaining pregnancy tissue. Cytotec is a prostaglandin, one of the hormones that initiate labor. Its use is discussed in detail under labor induction. It can be used to treat miscarriage and when doing so is given in doses ranging from two hundred to eight hundred micrograms placed vaginally or given orally. Cytotec causes the cervix to soften and the uterus muscle to contract. It frequently is all that is needed to result in completion of an incomplete miscarriage.

Second Trimester Pregnancy Loss

Over eighty percent of pregnancy loss occurs before twelve weeks gestation. However, approximately fifteen percent of clinically recognized pregnancy loss occurs in the second trimester. At least forty percent of pregnancies ending between twelve and twenty weeks have structural abnormalities incompatible with life.

Other than avoiding drugs, alcohol, and other teratogens (chemicals that cause birth defects), there is little you can do to prevent second trimester pregnancy loss. It is usually a baby that was developing with serious abnormalities, incompatible with life.

"Incompetent cervix" is a rare cause of pregnancy loss. It is shortening or dilating of the cervix *in the absence of uterine contractions*. Incompetent cervix is diagnosed if you've had at least one previous second trimester pregnancy loss of an apparently normal fetus in the absence of any other medical factor such as uterine infection, preterm labor, or placental abnormalities. "Incompetent cervix" is a diagnosis made "retrospectively" based on your past history and if you're having problems with your current pregnancy.

If your ob provider suspects incompetent cervix, she may perform an ultrasound to visually evaluate the cervix. If the cervix appears to be shortening without an explanation (examples above); your provider may recommend a "cerclage" to prevent pregnancy loss. A "cerclage" is a purse-string stitch around the cervix to reinforce it in the hope of preventing pregnancy loss. There is no firm evidence that cerclage prevents second trimester pregnancy loss, but it is sometimes done because there is nothing else that can be done.

Medications for preterm labor do not work for incompetent cervix. For one, the uterus lacks receptors for these medications in the second trimester. Second, incompetent cervix is believed to be caused by an intrinsically weak cervix, rather than uterine contractions or other factors.

Office Notes: Terry's Twins

One of the most rewarding parts of my job is the rare opportunity to perform miracles. Terry's Twins were a defining moment in my medical career and I will cherish their story forever.

I received a page from the emergency department physician at about one AM informing me he had a woman of twenty weeks gestation with twins. He stated it appeared the first twin was in the vagina, but the second twin was still in the uterus.

When I arrived to the Emergency Department I saw Terry and confirmed the E.R. doctor's assessment was correct. Both twins still had heart beats but it appeared inevitable Terry was going to lose the first twin, as she was already in the vagina on her way out of the body.

The twins had separate placentas and were in separate sacs (diamnionic, dichorionic).

I presented all the options to Terry and her husband, Phil: Allow nature to take its course and wait for the loss of both twins to occur spontaneously. The second option was to intervene and try to save the second twin by placing a cerclage in an attempt to prevent loss of the second twin.

I explained the chances of success were less than one percent—that the risk of breaking the second bag of waters during the procedure was high. I also advised Terry and Phil that even if we could save the second twin in the short term, it would be unlikely for that twin to survive to a viable gestational age; and that Terry would have to be at strict bed rest for the remainder of her pregnancy.

After discussing it among themselves Terry and Phil decided to proceed with option B and try to save the second twin.

We went back to the operating room. By the time we got there, the first twin had lost his heart beat and was born deceased. The second twin, however, was alive and well. I pushed that twin's bag of waters up as far into the cervix as I could and placed a cerclage. Terry and her twin did fine through the procedure.

However, I was not optimistic things would last. To my amazement, Terry and Twin B made it to twenty-eight weeks gestation—eight more weeks in utero. Terry came in to the birth place in active labor. She was too far advanced in labor to have time to transport her to a center with a "level III" nursery for extremely premature babies. Twin B delivered by C-section and was transported after birth to a neonatal intensive care unit. Terry recovered very well.

Twin B did well for a while, but eventually developed bronchopulmonary dysplasia, a serious lung complication of prematurity. She could not survive without a ventilator and expired at eight months of age.

Terry came into my office the day Twin B died and we held each other and cried together. She thanked me for all I did but I wasn't sure if it was for the best in the end. I couldn't know if Twin B suffered or felt pain; and if she did, I felt I was responsible for it.

Chapter 3

Hormones and Optimism: Ten to Twenty Weeks

You've made it through the first trimester and you begin to physically feel much better as you approach sixteen weeks gestation. Tremendous changes are taking place within, not just in fetal development, but in your hormone levels. Hormone levels have enormous impact on your physical, emotional, and mental well-being. This chapter will explore hormones in detail to help you understand why you're feeling what you're feeling.

In this chapter you will also learn more about fetal development and how to screen for genetic defects.

Hormones

Pregnancy is dominated by three major hormones, and several other minor ones. The "minor" hormones are still essential to pregnancy and abnormalities in any one of these hormones can lead to pregnancy loss. Each level of these hormones evolves dramatically as pregnancy progresses. The major hormones of pregnancy are estrogens, progesterone, and human chorionic gonadotropin (HCG). The minor ones are human placental lactogen (HPL) and fetal adrenal hormones.

> **Major Pregnancy Hormones:**
> - **Estrogens**
> - **Progesterone**
> - **Human Chorionic Gonadotropin (HCG)**
>
> **Minor Pregnancy Hormones:**
> - **Human Placental Lactogen (HPL)**
> - **Fetal Adrenal Hormones**

Estrogens

In the early weeks of pregnancy estrogen is produced by the mother's ovaries. However, by seven weeks gestation, the developing placenta becomes the major source of estrogen, and remains so throughout pregnancy. The major human estrogens are estradiol (most potent), estrone, and estriol.

At term the placenta produces so much estrogen, the mother is literally awash in a sea of estrogen. **The daily production of estrogen at term is equal to the total daily production of one thousand (1000) ovulating women.** Estrogen production is roughly proportional to the size of the placenta as the placenta is the primary source of estrogen throughout pregnancy.

Although the overall levels of estrogens increase steadily throughout pregnancy, at times they are made and released in a "pulsatile" fashion—or in packets, short bursts of hormones. Minute-to-minute changes in hormone levels occur and are responsible for the apparent "mood swings" so many pregnant women comment on.

> At term the daily production of estrogen at term is equal to the total daily production of one thousand (1000) ovulating women.

Physical Effects of Estrogens

Estrogens dilate blood vessels, increase ability of blood to clot, and increase levels of **endogenous endorphins** in the brain. Endogenous endorphins are opiate-like chemicals made naturally by the body. They are increased by exercise, estrogen and other hormones, and certain foods such as chocolate.

Estrogens improve nerve cell growth in the learning, memory, and emotional centers of the brain. Estrogens improve verbal memory and create a sense of well-being.

Estrogens can also cause nausea and breast tenderness. These hormones stimulate the growth and expansion of breast glands.

> **Some Effects of Estrogens**
> **Physical**
> - **Dilates blood vessels**
> - **Increases clotting**
> - **Breast Tenderness**
> - **Nausea**
>
> **Mental and Emotional**
> - **Increases hormones that regulate mood and thinking**
> - **Increases verbal memory**
> - **Increases "feel good" hormones**

Mental and Emotional Effects of Estrogens

By increasing endogenous endorphins estrogens can make you feel "high". Likewise, a sudden drop in estrogens leads to a drop in endogenous endorphins, and can cause a feeling of dysphoria (bad mood), irritability, and increase emotional outbursts.

Estrogens also increase serotonin levels in the brain. Serotonin is an important regulator of mood. Adjusment of serotonin levels is the mechanism of action of many pharmaceutical anti-depressants.

Estrogens increase the levels of a protein necessary to communicate memory and learning signals in the brain. Estrogen can give you a sense that you feel "smarter" and can concentrate better. This may be why many non-pregnant women feel better in the first half of their menstrual cycle—because that's when estrogen levels are increasing.

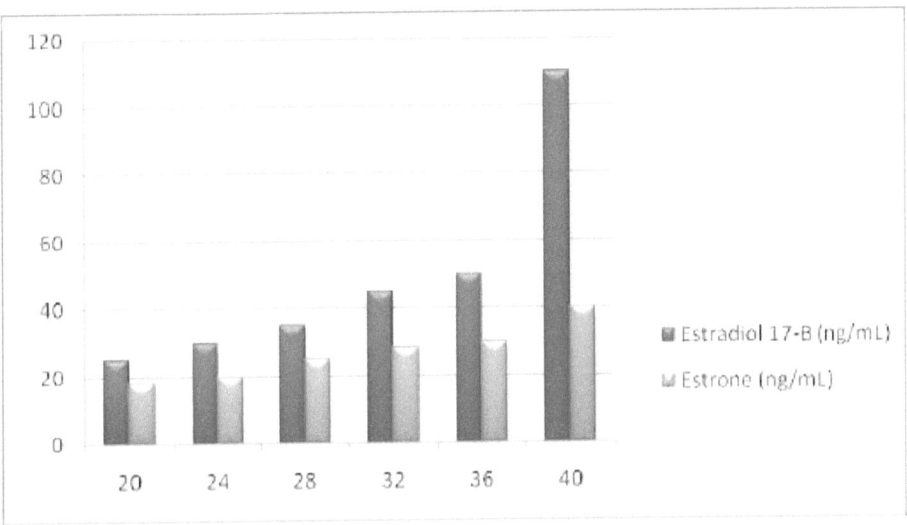

Estrogen levels throughout pregnancy. The weeks gestation is the horizontal axis and the hormone levels (in nanograms per milliliter) is the vertical axis. Both estradiol and estrone increase throughout pregnancy. Of these two estrogens, estradiol is the more potent. This bar graph was adapted from Cunningham, F. Gary *et al. Williams Obstetrics, 21ˢᵗ edition*, New York, McGraw Hill NY, 2001.

Progesterone

Progesterone and its related compounds, pregnenolone, allopregnenolone, and others undergo dramatic increases during pregnancy, similar to estrogen. Progesterones are also produced by the placenta and the fetal adrenal glands. Like estrogen, progesterone is synthesized and distributed in a pulsatile fashion.

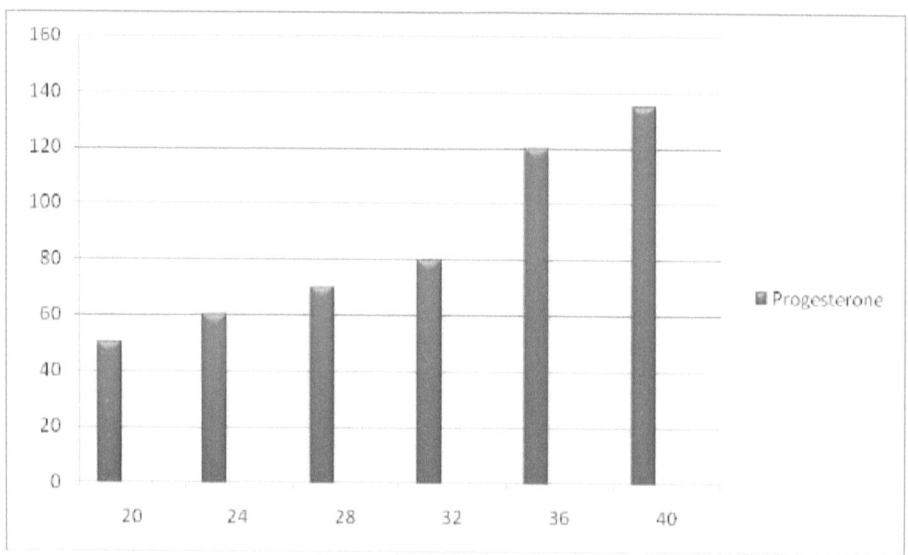

Progesterone levels throughout pregnancy. The weeks gestation is the horizontal axis and the progesterone level (in nanograms per milliliter) is the vertical axis. This bar graph was adapted from Cunningham, F. Gary *et al.* *Williams Obstetrics, 21st edition*, New York, McGraw Hill, 2001.

Physical Effects of Progesterone

Progesterone increases water retention, increases appetite, and can cause weight gain. Progesterone can affect blood pressure. It stimulates growth and expansion of breast glands, and can cause breast tenderness. Progesterone also causes a sensation of feeling short of breath. This is termed "dyspnea of pregnancy".

Mental and Emotional Effects of Progesterone and Related Hormones

A metabolic relative of progesterone, allopregnenolone (AP), interacts with GABA (gamma-alpha-butyric acid) receptors in the brain. The GABA system regulates anxiety levels and response to stress. Allopregnenolone (AP) increases the hormones that modulate the GABA system. It therefore eases anxiety and increases capacity to manage stress.

AP has been shown to be low in women who suffer from post-partum depression and premenstrual syndrome, compared to women who do not suffer these disorders.

> **Some Effects of Progesterone**
> **Physical**
> - **Breast Swelling and Tenderness**
> - **Weight Gain**
> - **Melasma (Darkening of facial skin)**
> - **Shortness of Breath**
>
> **Mental and Emotional**
> - **Sleepiness**
> - **Anxiety suppression**
> - **Stress reduction**

Progesterone can be sedating, induce relaxation, relieve anxiety and irritability, and help with response to stress. Sudden drops in progesterone as with childbirth or onset of menses in non-pregnant women can cause irritability, anxiety, and feeling depressed.

Progesterone increases throughout pregnancy but undergoes a prominent upswing beginning at twenty weeks. This is when many women report onset of "progesterone headaches". Once women accommodate to the high levels of progesterone the headaches stop, usually by twenty-six weeks or sooner.

Human Chorionic Gonadotrophin (HCG)

HCG is the quintessential "pregnancy hormone": the one the pregnancy tests measure. The placenta makes the majority of HCG; but a small percentage is synthesized by the fetal adrenal glands. Unlike other pregnancy hormones which gradually increase throughout preg-

> **Effects of HCG:**
> - **Fatigue**
> - **Nausea**
> - **Breast Tenderness**

nancy, HCG shoots up and peaks at twelve weeks then drops to minimal levels, followed by a very slow rise to term. However, HCG levels never again approach their twelve-weeks status.

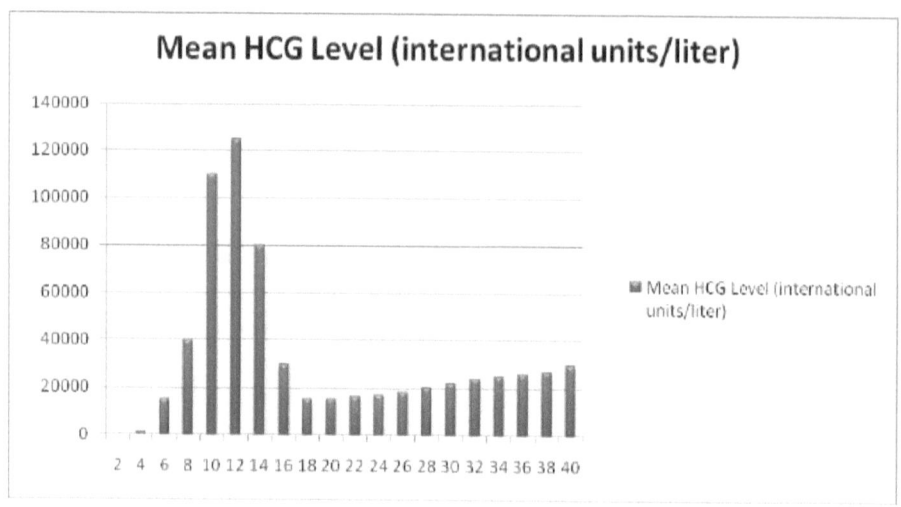

Mean HCG levels in pregnancy expressed as international units/liter per weeks gestation from two to forty. HCG doubles every 48 hours in early pregnancy, peaks at 10-12 weeks, then drops and rises slowly thereafter. This bar graph was adapted from Gabbe, Steven G., *et al. Obstetrics: Normal and Problem Pregnancies*. New York, Churchill, Livingstone. 1996.

HCG is responsible for the first trimester "blahs": nausea, fatigue, lack of energy, and wanting to sleep all the time. As HCG levels drop between twelve and sixteen weeks, energy level increases and you feel that second trimester "bloom". HCG is made by the early embryo and can be detected emerging from six- to eight-cell sized embryos.

HCG probably enters the maternal blood stream when the embryo implants into the uterine wall. It is detectable seven to eight days after fertilization. However, due to the variability in time between onset of menses and ovulation, early HCG levels should not cause undue concern, unless they are not rising appropriately. Between fertilization and twelve weeks of pregnancy HCG levels roughly double every forty-eight hours. However normal pregnancies may show as little as a thirty percent and as much as a sixty percent increase in HCG levels in any given forty-eight hour period.

Serial HCG levels are often used by medical practitioners to determine if a pregnancy is normal or not. HCG levels in conjunction with ultrasound can be used to diagnose miscarriage and ectopic pregnancy (pregnancy outside the uterus).

HCG is now being used in "first trimester serum" screening for Down's syndrome and other chromosomal defects. HCG is often abnormal in abnormal pregnancies. This hormone level, in conjunction with ultrasound can be used as early as 10-1/2 to 11-1/2 weeks gestation to identify major genetic defects and other lethal problems.

> **Utility of HCG**
> - **Distinguishing normal from abnormal pregnancy**
> - **Diagnosing miscarriage and ectopic pregnancy**
> - **Detecting serious genetic defects**

HCG structurally resembles other hormones such as thyroid stimulating hormone (TSH), luteinizing hormone (the ovulation hormone—LH), and adrenal corticotrophin (ACTH). Tests for HCG can cross-react with some of these other hormones, particularly the ovulation hormone, LH.

Fetal Adrenal Glands and Hormones

The fetal adrenal glands are important "middle actors" in production of most pregnancy hormones. The fetal adrenal glands make proteins necessary for conversion of some hormones from inactive precursor states to active states. They also make precursors for some pregnancy hormones. There is a complex interplay between the fetal adrenal glands, the placenta, and the maternal hormone production centers in the brain and ovaries. A normal fetus is essential for normal production of many pregnancy hormones.

The fetal adrenal glands may also play a role in the onset of labor. There is evidence the fetus sends a "maturity" signal to the mother's body, and is responsible, in large part, for initiating labor.

Importance of Cholesterol

Cholesterol is an essential ingredient in many pregnancy hormones and for adrenal hormones that modulate response to stress. Cholesterol cannot be made by the body so it is crucial to obtain it from the food you eat.

The fetal brain also requires cholesterol and other fats to develop.

Pregnancy is not the time for a low fat diet, but for a well balanced diet that includes vegetables, "healthy" fats (liquid at room temperature), a few eggs and some ice cream. Everything in moderation is key.

Other Hormones

Human Placental Lactogen (HPL) is produced by the placenta and structurally resembles growth hormone and prolactin (the milk-producing hormone). HPL is synthesized by the placenta and regulates maternal metabolism. It is responsible for shifting nutrients consumed by mom to the baby. HPL also can interfere with maternal insulin. Gestational diabetes is related to excess maternal weight gain, in part by the increased placental volume and increased production of HPL.

Relaxin

Ahh … wouldn't life be nice if we could all just take some "relaxin" when we're feeling stressed? Actually relaxin is a hormone produced by the placenta and uterus. It acts on uterine muscle cells to prevent contractions. It doesn't relieve stress … oh well.

> **Cholesterol and other fats are crucial for fetal brain development and pregnancy hormone production.**

Second Trimester Physical Symptoms

Round Ligament Pain

Round ligament pain is one of the most common reasons for phone calls to ob providers and unscheduled prenatal visits in the second trimester. It is caused by growth and stretching of the ligaments supporting the uterus in the pelvis. Round ligament pain usually starts around sixteen weeks and eases off after twenty weeks.

It can be a sharp pain that doubles you over. It can occur anywhere from the belly button area down to the labia and inner thigh. You may think you have appendicitis. Sometimes it is so severe it leads to dizziness and nausea.

Round ligament pain can occur spontaneously or it can be triggered by changes in position and walking. It responds to rest, acetaminophen (Tylenol), and a mildly warm heating pad (lowest setting). A lukewarm bath also relieves round ligament pain. If you have pain that doesn't respond to these measures, or pain accompanied by fever, nausea, and vomiting you should quickly seek medical attention.

Bleeding and Spotting

Second trimester spotting is common and most of the time does not signify there is a problem. However, bright red bleeding can be the sign of a cervix infection, a placental problem, or other problems. Ongoing bright red bleeding should prompt you to seek medical attention.

Energy Level

Parallel to HCG levels, your energy usually reaches a low point at twelve weeks. At twelve weeks you're often wondering, "Why did I do this? What was I thinking?" You may even feel a bit depressed. These emotions have physical reasons behind them—hormone changes and their effects on your energy level. If you can ride it out with extra sleep, relaxation, and exercise, you'll usually feel better by sixteen to twenty weeks. If you do not feel better, consult your ob provider as you may have pregnancy-related depression.

After twelve weeks, energy gradually improves as HCG drops until about twenty weeks. The mid-second trimester is when most people feel best. You may have an "excess" amount of energy, begin projects, and engage in other activities to expend your energy. If you're feeling anxious a walk is one of the best cures—forty-five minutes on flat ground. Take water to drink.

Interest in sex increases as HCG drops and estrogen and progesterone become more dominant. For one thing, you're usually not exhausted all the time.

Beyond twenty weeks, energy levels are more variable and susceptible to external factors such as work, whether you have other young children, and other issues not related to pregnancy. However, the physical changes in your body can magnify the impact of these external factors on your energy level. The excess weight, strain on your muscles, bones, and joints can make you fatigue with less effort than usual. Toward term you may experience fluctuations in energy level associated with sleep disturbance and late pregnancy physical changes.

Appetite Changes

Appetite varies from person to person. Generally it increases around twenty weeks, especially if you had nausea in the first trimester. It is not unusual for people to lose a few pounds in the first trimester between nausea, pregnancy ambivalence, and food aversions or cravings.

One way to alleviate nausea and control weight gain is to eat small frequent meals (about five per day) throughout pregnancy. Remember fats are brain food for you and the baby. Don't overdo it, but they are an essential part of your diet.

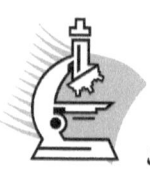

Science Notes: Second trimester embryology and fetal movement

By fourteen weeks gestation all the fetal cells have migrated to their positions and the major organs have been formed. From this point on most of the organs are maturing by adding on new cells, growing existing cells, and establishing metabolic pathways to function.

The second trimester is the brain trimester. A good part of the cerebral cortex (the thinking part of the brain) grows and develops during the second trimester. Nerve cells are added and mature. Chemical connections are made and enriched. Fats, cholesterol, proteins, and other nutrients are essential to brain development.

Fetal movement can be seen as early as eight weeks on ultrasound. As the nervous system matures, spontaneous signals pass along the nerves to stimulate muscle growth. We don't know exactly when fetuses "hear" but second trimester fetuses do move in response to acoustic-vibration stimulation. This can be seen on ultrasound as early as twelve to fourteen weeks.

However, most women don't feel the fetus move until after sixteen weeks. This isn't because the fetus is not moving; rather it is small relative to the fluid volume and uterus so the movements are "buffered" by the fluid and not perceived by the mom.

It is known that the eyelids are fused shut until twenty-two to twenty-four weeks gestation. The fetus is not "blind" but early vision is probably "fuzzy".

Early Genetic Screening and Testing: What should you do and when?

A **screening test** is often confused with a **diagnostic test**. A screening test is designed to predict the likelihood of a condition, while a diagnostic test confirms the presence or absence of a condition. A Pap smear is a screening test for cervical cancer, while a biopsy (tissue sample) of the cervix is a diagnostic test for cervical cancer. Some tests, such as cholesterol levels, serve both screening and diagnostic purposes.

Pregnancy screening tests are: ultrasound and maternal serum screening in the first and/or second trimester. **Pregnancy diagnostic tests** are: ultrasound, amniocentesis, and chorionic villus sampling.

> **Pregnancy screening tests:**
> - **Ultrasound**
> - **Serum Screening**
>
> **Pregnancy diagnostic tests:**
> - **Amniocentesis**
> - **Chorionic Villus Sampling**
> - **Ultrasound**

In considering whether or not to undergo any of these tests you should decide what you will do with the test results. Many people are satisfied with the risk prediction of pregnancy screening tests, even though they are aware these tests cannot definitively diagnose a condition. This can sometimes be misleading as a small percentage of screening tests are wrong.

Pregnancy screening tests (discussed below) are intended for low-risk populations of women under age thirty-five. If you're thirty-five or over your ob provider will probably offer you the definitive test, amniocentesis or chorionic villus sampling (placental tissue sampling). You can opt for or decline any test offered but do not take offense at being offered the test, as ob providers are held to a standard of care, an element of which is offering screening and diagnostic tests for genetic disorders based on known risk factors. Some tests are recommended as elements of managing pregnancy and delivery.

The age, thirty-five, is used as a cut-off for recommending diagnostic pregnancy tests because that is the age at which the risk of the test is lower than the risk of a chromosomal or other serious birth defect. As you approach age forty the risk of a chromosomal defect reaches two percent and shoots up thereafter.

Nuchal Translucency and Early Ultrasound

Many serious genetic defects can be detected with ultrasound in the first trimester. As the resolution of ultrasound has improved we've learned a great deal about mid-trimester fetal anatomy.

Many major birth defects cause problems with the heart, nervous system, and fetal circulatory system (of blood and lymph fluid). These defects lead to accumulation of fluid in the skin behind the neck. This area is on ultrasound is identified as the "nuchal translucency". Nuchal translucency done at eleven weeks can detect Down's syndrome, serious heart defects, and other chromosomal problems. It is often combined with "serum screening" (measurement of proteins in the maternal blood) to predict the risk of birth defects.

Nuchal translucency is the measurement of the dark area between the fetal spine and the fetal skin at the back of the neck. It changes with gestational age and is most useful if done between 10-1/2 and 11-1/2 weeks. It can be done up to 13-1/2 weeks but becomes less accurate as gestational age advances.

Nuchal translucency alone can detect sixty to eighty percent of Down's syndrome and other serious chromosomal abnormalities. Many defects seen at eleven weeks are not compatible with life; they are either serious heart defects or extra or missing chromosomes. Many fetuses with very abnormal nuchal translucencies do not survive pregnancy.

However, nuchal translucency is highly variable and dependent upon technology and human error. A national certification program exists to establish competency and conduct ongoing quality control regarding nuchal translucency.

First Trimester Serum Screening

First trimester serum screening is relatively new as of 2008 and it is being offered to varying degrees in the United States. It is often done in conjunction with or instead of nuchal translucency. First trimester screening is sometimes restricted to areas with access to chorionic villus sampling (CVS), the first trimester diagnostic chromosomal test.

First trimester serum screening involves measuring proteins in maternal blood: human chorionic gonadotropin (HCG), and pregnancy-associated-plasma-protein-A (PAPP-A). First trimester serum screening is combined with nuchal translucency measurements to obtain the highest detection rates for Down's syndrome (about eighty-five percent).

These values are compared with normal ranges for gestational age and maternal age to arrive at a risk factor for genetic defects. A condition can only be predicted, not confirmed with first trimester screening. Confirmation requires a chromosome test such as amniocentesis or chronionic villus sampling.

Second Trimester Serum Screening (Maternal Serum Quad Screen)

Second trimester serum screening involves measuring four proteins in maternal blood: human chorionic gonadotropin (HCG), alpha-fetoprotein (AFP), estriol, and inhibin. It is done at fifteen to twenty weeks gestation and predicts eighty-five percent of babies with Down's syndrome. The quad screen can also predict the risks of neural tube defects (spina bifida), and other chromosomal problems besides Down's syndrome.

The quad screen is widely available and offered to all women thirty-five and under.

Mid-Trimester Ultrasound

Second trimester ultrasound is often done at sixteen to twenty weeks gestation. Ultrasound does not harm the baby. However, a large study on ultrasound done in the early 1990's (called the RADIUS trial) showed that screening mid-trimester ultrasound in *low risk* women does not decrease fetal or neonatal mortality rates.

Although screening ultrasound has not been proven to be of benefit (at least with 1990's technology), most people expect ultrasound. If the RADIUS trial were repeated today, with modern equipment and personnel, and with the training received in a typical obstetrics-gynecology residency, the results may be different (or not).

Diagnostic ultrasound is useful in evaluating specific problems. Some heart defects can be better evaluated and defined with ultrasound. Other anatomic defects such as spina bifida and abdominal wall defects can be identified with ultrasound. Some chromosomal defects, including some cases of Down's syndrome, can be detected with ultrasound. However, fifty percent of Down's babies appear normal at a twenty weeks ultrasound scan.

Amniocentesis

Amniocentesis ("amnio") is obtaining fetal chromosomes from amniotic fluid to diagnose Down's syndrome and other genetic conditions. Amnio is done between fifteen and twenty weeks' gestation. Amnio earlier than fifteen weeks carries a risk of causing limb defects, but is very safe after fifteen weeks. Amniocentesis has a pregnancy loss rate of roughly 1/1000 in most contemporary U.S. centers.

Amnio is recommended when you're thirty-five years of age or older; or if you have an abnormal first or second trimester screen. Amnio is widely available throughout the United States. Definitive results can sometimes take up to ten days so it is wise to do amnio as early as possible.

Chorionic Villus Sampling (CVS)

CVS requires more training and skill than amniocentesis and is not widely available in the United States. In some states there may be no one or just one or two people qualified to do CVS. Usually these people are employed at medical schools.

CVS involves sampling the placenta via the cervix or through the abdominal wall to obtain fetal chromosomes. Some CVS results can be available as early as one day, but definitive results usually take about a week.

CVS has a miscarriage rate of roughly one percent. It has the distinct advantage of being available in the first trimester (best done at eleven weeks); whereas amniocentesis is not available until the second trimester.

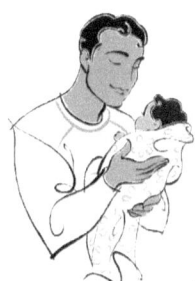

For Dads: Intercourse and Mood Changes

If you comprehend hormones you may have a better understanding of the mother of your baby. You know her hormones are all over the map. First she's tired for three months; then if you're lucky she becomes a sex-crazed love goddess by about sixteen weeks. Enjoy it because after baby there's no sex for at least six weeks, and sometimes longer.

Sex drive in women is much more vulnerable than in men to external factors like work hours, stress, and the presence of small children. If your honey's not in the mood don't push it as it will only stress her more as you're adding to her never ending "to do" list. (Yes, she really views it that way).

There's a lot you can do to get show your honey you care and it doesn't involve buying flowers. Do the laundry. Vacuum the floors. Clean the bathrooms. These will make her feel loved and turn your woman on; and be more likely to elicit the desired response than flowers, chocolate, or possibly even diamonds.

Chapter 4

Viability: Twenty to Twenty-Six Weeks

Late in the second, early in the third trimester your pregnancy goes from being an abstract entity to a tangible being. You may know the gender of your baby. She may have a room. He may have a name. You probably have his first few days of clothes arranged on his bed. You've distributed ultrasound pictures to your friends and family and you may have even started an album.

Definitions

Viability

Pregnancy viability is the time at which a fetus can live independently outside the womb. This occurs at about twenty-four weeks' gestation, but some factors can push this earlier or later in specific instances. There is evidence that maternal physical and mental stress speeds fetal lung maturity. For example, if your water breaks early or if you have a history of preterm labor, your baby's lungs may be mature enough for the baby to survive outside your body at an earlier age than your pregnant friend who hasn't experienced these stressors.

The definition of viability is roughly equivalent to survivability and is the opposite of mortality, which is the rate of fetal or neonatal demise. The percentage of mortality decreases drastically with gestational age from fifty percent at twenty-six weeks to a fraction of a percent by thirty-two weeks' gestation.

Viability differs from morbidity. Morbidity is a medical term describing the effects of an illness or state of being. Morbidity is the consequences or complications of an illness or treatment. For example, the morbidities of prematurity include brain damage, inability to breathe adequately, inability to digest milk, and inability to maintain a stable temperature. Morbidity also drops dramatically between twenty-six and thirty-two weeks' gestational age.

Preterm Birth

Preterm birth is defined as birth occurring at less than thirty-seven weeks completed gestation or birth of a baby weighing less than 2500 grams. However,

> **Preterm birth: You have more control than you realize.**

most serious consequences of early birth occur in babies born less than thirty-two weeks gestation and weighing less than 1500 grams.

Incidence

The incidence of preterm birth in the United States hasn't changed substantially since the 1960s. It remains about eight to ten percent of all births and it has actually increased slightly since the 1960s. While a fixed percentage of preterm birth is not preventable (no one knows exactly what that percentage is), some preterm birth is dependent on mom's behavior during pregnancy and can be prevented. One of my goals in this book is to make you aware you have a great deal of control over prevention of preterm birth of your baby. We can decrease the rate of preterm birth, one mother at a time, if we take care of ourselves and observe habits discussed in this chapter.

Gestational age and Survival

What *has* changed is survivability. Advances in technology have increased the survival rate of premature infants. Greater than thirty-two weeks gestation, there is little difference between survival rates with no permanent impairments, among these and infants born at term. The greatest variability occurs with infants born in the twenty-six to twenty-eight week range.

Complications of prematurity decrease progressively in the twenty-eight to thirty-two week range. Infants born at less than twenty-eight weeks have much higher rates of brain abnormalities resulting from bleeding in the head, immature lungs and digestive systems; and are much more susceptible to the impact of infection and nutritional factors than infants born over twenty-eight weeks gestation. "Cerebral palsy" (defined below) is much more closely correlated with gestational age and weight at birth than with factors occurring during delivery.

These complications of prematurity tend to decrease in jumps rather than in a linear fashion. For example blindness, lung disease, and cerebral palsy are very high in infants born at twenty-six weeks. However these problems drop at twenty-eight weeks and plummet to the low percentile range at thirty-two weeks. Babies born at thirty-two weeks or greater in the "developed" world have very few complications of prematurity with modern technology. While babies born at thirty-six weeks and beyond are considered "full term" as far as morbidity and mortality are concerned.

Gestational age is a guideline for survival but it cannot be relied upon without question. Some twenty-six-weekers have no problems whatsoever, while some twenty-eight or thirty week babies have debilitating complications and ultimately succumb to these.

There are certain limits of nature which are insurmountable. With rare exceptions, a baby's lungs, brain, and other organs simply aren't developed enough before twenty-four weeks gestation for most babies to survive outside the uterus. How much to invest in rescuing a premature fetus depends on the consequences. Some extremely premature babies are rescued only to sit in a vegetative state in a nursery, hooked up to a ventilator, never to

> **Risk Factors for Preterm Birth:**
> - **Poor Maternal Weight Gain**
> - **Over-work and Stress**
> - **Prior Preterm Birth**
> - **Bleeding During Pregnancy**
> - **High Blood Pressure**
> - **Diabetes**
> - **Drug and Alcohol Use**
> - **Tobacco Use**
> - **Poor dental hygiene**
> - **Infection**
> - **Multiple sex partners**
> - **Lack of self-care**
> - **Placental problems**
> - **Medical illnesses**
> - **Multiple gestations (twins, etc.)**

know consciousness; only to expire after a few months or years in this state. Is that a humane thing to do to a living being? I realize these are subjective moral questions that only you can decide for yourself for your specific circumstances. However, I implore you to consider the line between salvation and torture. In the twenty-three to twenty-five week range this line can be a hair thin.

My heart goes out to you if you're faced with delivering an extremely premature baby. You must consider the opinions of your neonatologist (doctor who specializes in premature babies) and obstetrician, but the ultimate decisions are up to you and any higher power in which you believe.

Preterm Birth: Prevention and Recognition

Some causes of preterm birth are not preventable. These include natural multiple gestations, placental problems, prior preterm birth, and certain medical illnesses (see box).

> **Preterm labor = contractions + cervical change.**

However, many preventable causes of preterm birth have been identified. You can prevent preterm birth by being healthy before you become pregnant. This means refraining from using tobacco, illegal drugs, and alcohol. Maintain a normal weight prior to pregnancy and follow the weight gain guidelines in Chapter One. Minimize your exposure to infection by remaining monogamous. Brush your teeth! It decreases the risk of infection and preterm birth. (Do I sound like your mother?) Avoid over-working and excess stress. Develop your own reliable stress management tools. Exercise in moderation—walking forty-five minutes daily is excellent pregnancy exercise (unless you're having preterm contractions).

Risk Factors for Preterm Birth

Risk factors for preterm birth include over-work (being on your feet more than eight hours per day); illegal drug and tobacco use, bleeding during pregnancy, the extremes of maternal age (being under fifteen or over thirty-five), placental problems, and medical illnesses such as diabetes, high blood pressure, and other complications of pregnancy. Sex does not cause preterm birth but it can aggravate preterm contractions if you're having serious contractions, and it can trigger vaginal bleeding. Dehydration and exhaustion can cause a bout of preterm contractions. I often see people for preterm contractions on hot summer days after they've over-exerted themselves physically e.g. moving or painting the baby's room. Rest often. Listen to your body if it's telling you you're tired. Drink plenty of water.

Recognizing Symptoms of Preterm Labor

Preterm labor is defined as contractions before thirty-seven weeks gestation *that produce changes in the cervix.* Cervical change (thinning, shortening, softening, or dilation of the cervix) is

> **Contractions are frequently felt in the evening.**

essential to meet the criteria for preterm labor. Literally every woman has preterm contractions. These are normal and are called "Braxton Hicks" contractions (BHC's). BHC's are usually non-painful but can sometimes feel like infrequent menstrual cramps. You will have BHC's during your pregnancy. They are triggered by the uterus growing and hormonal changes of pregnancy. It is not uncommon to have four to six BHC's per hour, especially during the evening hours of six to eleven PM. However, if you are having BHC's that are sustained and becoming painful you need medical attention. In fact, most BHC's, preterm contractions, false labor, and real labor begins between these hours of the evening. There is a "circadian" or daily pattern to contraction hormones, leading to more frequent contractions in the evening and night time hours.

BHC's increase with gestational age and with the number of babies you've had. If you've had one or two babies before, you usually experience BHC's earlier on in pregnancy and with greater frequency.

Having had two preterm labors myself, I know what preterm labor feels like compared to BHC's. Preterm labor contractions tend to be more painful, are felt lower down in the abdomen "like severe menstrual cramps" and usually increase in frequency and severity over a few hours. Preterm labor contractions can go away with rest and drinking water. So can BHC's.

Preterm labor can feel like back pain or pelvic pressure. You may also just feel like you have the "flu" and have no abdominal or pelvic symptoms.

It can be very difficult to differentiate between preterm labor and BHC's, especially in the twenty-three to twenty-six week range, so if you have any question about the sensations you're experiencing, consult your healthcare provider, or go to the hospital. If you telephone your provider don't be surprised if she instructs you to go into the hospital for evaluation because preterm labor cannot be diagnosed or ruled out over the phone.

Round Ligament Pain or Contractions?

> **If it's sharp and sudden think round ligament pain.**

The difference between round ligament pain and contractions is round ligament pain is sharp and sudden (it can be so sharp you need to sit or lie down—you may feel like you have something serious like appendicitis!). Round ligament pain usually comes on suddenly, is triggered by movement or a change in position, and typically resolves within ten minutes of lying down. On the other hand, contractions are usually crampy rather than sharp, are rhythmic; and have a gradual onset.

Round ligament pain is caused by stretching of the ligaments that support the uterus in the pelvis and it can be brought on by moving or standing for prolonged time periods.

Round ligament pain also responds to a mild heating pad and acetaminophen (Tylenol); whereas preterm labor does not.

Round ligament pain usually begins at about sixteen weeks gestation, is episodic, intermittent, and often (but not always) goes away by twenty-six weeks of gestation.

Diagnosis of Preterm Labor

Diagnosis of preterm labor requires a cervical exam, ultrasound or other assessment of your cervix. Go to the hospital if you think you have preterm labor. At the hospital the nurses or ob providers will put you on the monitor to see if you're having contractions. Your cervix will also be checked unless you have a medical reason for not having a cervical exam (such as placenta previa). Over eighty percent of people who come to the hospital to be evaluated for preterm labor do not actually have preterm labor. Rather, they have preterm contractions not leading to cervical change, Braxton Hicks contractions, or some other problem.

It can be impossible to distinguish preterm labor from BHC's and false labor. The only reliable way to differentiate these conditions is to have a medical evaluation. If you have any doubt you should seek medical attention.

Early Symptoms Change

Many symptoms discussed in Chapters Three and Four evolve throughout the late second and early third trimester. These are summarized below.

o **Energy Level:** Usually increases at twenty weeks, lasts until about thirty-two weeks then starts to decrease again; affected by sleep and stress.

o **Appetite changes, reflux:** Cravings change throughout pregnancy. What was once appetizing can invoke thoughts of projectile vomiting. As the baby grows it presses on your abdomen, stomach, and ribs. This can cause indigestion. Over-the-counter antacids are safe and work well for indigestion.

o **Emotional State:** Two words: "Roller Coaster". One minute you can be level, even, then euphoric, and then crying. This is called "emotional lability". You may feel like you're going crazy but it's really your hormones. Pregnancy hormones are powerful and they are produced in a pulsatile fashion (short bursts) rather than in nice steady even levels. This accounts for rapid flip-flops from one emotional state to another. Emotional lability may produce anxiety because you don't understand it and can't control it. If you're feeling anxious try relaxation techniques such as abdominal breathing, progressive muscle relaxation, and going for a walk. If you can, try to "neutralize" your emotional state, especially if you find yourself "out of control". A technique to neutralize your emotions is to remind yourself they are temporary and will pass. Are you feeling "reactionary"? If so, try to establish the cause and "think" your way through it. If your husband gives you that look that tells you he thinks you've lost your mind, remind him to read and re-read this book, especially chapters three, this one, and the chapter for dads.

o   ***Sciatica/Back pain:*** As the baby grows, the uterus presses on your back muscles and sciatic nerve. It also fills the pelvis. This can cause low back pain, lordosis (sway back), sciatica (pain that runs down the back of your leg); and pressure on the pubic bone, hip bones, and lower spine. All of these are uncomfortable but trust me, you will survive them all and almost everything will improve … after you deliver. These aches and pains respond to yoga, back stretches ("cat" stretches), rest, and relaxation techniques.

o   ***Constipation:*** The pregnancy hormone, progesterone, slows down your intestines as gestational age progresses. This results in constipation. It is crucial to drink water (about a gallon or more per day) to avoid constipation. If you live in a dry climate, it's summertime, or you exercise you need to drink more water. You can safely use stool softeners in pregnancy (docusate sodium) but avoid laxatives which may stimulate intestinal motility as these can also cause uterine contractions.

o   ***Sleep Changes:*** Every pregnant woman has insomnia. There are a number of causes: excitement, anticipation, worry, hormone changes, hot flashes, and concerns about the baby being normal. Marital stress often occurs during pregnancy and can worsen insomnia. It is crucial to treat insomnia—don't ignore it—because sleep deprivation decreases your overall health, immune system, and makes you more emotional. Sleep deprivation actually harms the logic part of the brain (the frontal lobe) and makes the emotion centers (amygdala, hippocampus) hyperactive. Sleep deprivation anytime, but especially in pregnancy, decreases your ability to respond to day-to-day stressors. In addition to affecting your emotional state and thinking processes, sleep can trigger or worsen preterm labor.

o   ***Sex:*** Sex changes throughout pregnancy. Different couples have varying comfort levels with sex. Sex is safe at any gestational age. It may become more uncomfortable as things progress and you may need to adjust with position changes and other measures. Fatigue exerts more influence later in pregnancy.

o   ***Shortness of Breath:*** As the baby grows it pushes upward on your lungs and reduces the volume of air you can take with each breath. The hormone, progesterone, also gives you a sensation that you're short of breath (termed "dyspnea of pregnancy"). Focus on taking five abdominal breaths when you're feeling particularly short of breath. This sensation will resolve after delivery.

Treatments for preterm birth

Some of the best treatments for preterm birth are not medications. Bed-rest, stress reduction, and relaxation exercises do wonders for alleviating preterm contractions. In the event of real preterm labor, your health care provider may use a number of treatments to stop contractions and mitigate the risks of early delivery.

No medication has been shown to reduce the rate of preterm birth. The best they can do is to delay birth until measures can be taken to reduce the consequences of preterm birth.

Every day in the womb is worth three in the neonatal intensive care unit (NICU). We want to keep those babies in the womb as long as circumstances will allow. We can optimize the tragedy of premature birth by administering drugs to slow preterm labor long enough for drugs that stimulate lung maturity, and protect the baby to take effect.

Medications to Stop Contractions

Terbutaline

Terbutaline is a beta agonist—it stimulates a receptor on the uterus muscle that produces relaxation of the uterus. It is effective for delaying delivery up to forty-eight hours but it does not reduce the incidence of preterm delivery. Terbutaline has been used to treat preterm labor since the 1960's. It is very safe, but not entirely without side effects. It can increase your heart rate, make you feel short of breath; and if you're diabetic it can cause problems regulating your sugar.

Terbutaline is short-acting and processed quickly by the body. It has no known ill effects on babies.

Magnesium Sulfate

Magnesium sulfate is a muscle relaxant. It lowers blood pressure and dilates your blood vessels. It also may delay but not prevent preterm delivery. It has been in use since the 1980's and has no known permanent adverse effects on babies.

Magnesium sulfate can make you feel sedated, short of breath, flushed, and generally uncomfortable. Magnesium sulfate can make it feel difficult for you to move like you're a "noodle'. It is administered as a continuous intravenous infusion and is metabolized quickly by the body.

Nifedipine

Nifedipine is a calcium channel blocker (muscle relaxant), that was originally developed to treat high blood pressure. Nifedipine is given by mouth and can cause side effects similar to magnesium sulfate. The predominant side effect of Nifedipine is headache and low blood pressure. It is usually not used in combination with magnesium sulfate for this reason. However, certain clinical circumstances such as very early and refractory preterm labor may dictate simultaneous use of multiple medications if the benefits outweigh the risks.

Indocin, Sulindac

Indocin and Sulindac are prostaglandin synthetase inhibitors (similar to ibuprofen). They work at a different molecular level than the other drugs to stop or prevent contractions. This class of drugs cannot be used after thirty-two weeks gestation, nor can they be used longer than seventy-two hours due to risk of fetal circulation complications and reduction of amniotic fluid volume. They are very safe and effective when used appropriately. They may cause stomach upset, but tend to have fewer maternal side effects than the other drugs.

Betamethasone

Betamethasone is a corticosteroid that is given to enhance fetal lung maturity in the event of an impending (within twenty-four hours) preterm birth. It is administered as a set of two injections twelve to twenty-four hours apart. It acts in a short period of time to accelerate lung maturity, minimize respiratory distress, and reduce intraventricular hemorrhage and other sequelae of premature birth. A course of betamethasone is only used between twenty-four to thirty-four weeks gestation and the benefits last for about one week. It is usually not repeated because there is no proven benefit to repeated doses.

Antibiotics

Penicillins are given in cases of imminent preterm birth to prevent an infection called "Group B Strep" sepsis or pneumonia. Preterm babies are at high risk for this infection due to their partially developed immune systems.

Consequences for Newborns of Preterm Birth

All these medications can be used in the hopes of preventing life-altering consequences of prematurity. These include:

Thermal Instability: Premies have difficulty maintaining normal body temperature and are at higher risk for infection.

Intraventricular Hemorrhage: The vessel membranes in premies' heads are unstable and they can easily bleed into the spinal fluid spaces of the brain. This can sometimes result in permanent brain damage, cerebral palsy, or learning disabilities.

Respiratory Distress and Brochopulmonary Dysplasia: Initial respiratory distress can be alleviated with a medication called surfactant which improves the expansion of the small lung sacs (alveoli). The underdeveloped lungs of premies present long-term challenges to simply obtain oxygen. Chronic treatment for lung immaturity and chronic oxygen therapy can result in bronchopulmonary dysplasia. This condition arises when microscopic changes occur in the alveoli (microscopic breathing sacs) of the lungs causing permanent lung "stiffness" and respiratory disease.

Necrotizing Enterocolitis (NEC): NEC means the intestines lack the maturity to process food normally. They can actually bleed, lose sheaves of surface lining, and increase susceptibility to life-threatening intestinal infection. The incidence of NEC is reduced a few percentage points by the use of betamethasone for imminent preterm birth, but steroids do not completely prevent NEC.

Retinopathy of Prematurity: Abnormal vessels of the retina which develop under abnormal oxygen and maturity environments. It can cause poor eyesight long term, and even blindness.

Cerebral Palsy (CP): Cerebral palsy is defined by the National Institutes of Health as a "non progressive motor disorder of early infant onset involving one or more limbs, with resulting muscular spasticity or paralysis".

Extensive research on cerebral palsy has shown premature birth is the single strongest risk factor for cerebral palsy. However, a risk factor is not inevitability. The incidence of cerebral palsy is about 1.5/1000 births and it has remained fairly stable for the past century, despite the advent of fetal monitoring during labor, increased cesarean deliveries, and improvements in obstetric care. In fact, the incidence of CP seems to be increasing slightly with the increased survival rates of infants born before thirty-two weeks gestation.

There is so much we do not understand about the human brain and nerve development that one infant born at twenty-six weeks may be totally normal, while another may be quadriplegic and developmentally delayed (have severe cerebral palsy).

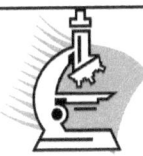

Science Notes: Periventricular Malacia, Prematurity, and Cerebral Palsy

Periventricular Malacia is a phenomenon found often in the brains of premature infants in which there is loss of brain matter around the "ventricles" (spinal fluid spaces) as well as within the major nerve mass of the brain. Twenty to one hundred percent of infants with ultrasonographic evidence of periventricular malacia have varying degrees of cerebral palsy (CP).

Periventricular malacia is associated with poor myelination (development of nerve insulation protein) and appears to have many causes, most of which occur before or during early pregnancy. CP is strongly associated with prematurity; although there are other risk factors:

➤ Risk Factors for CP Preceding Pregnancy
  o Women with long intervals between periods
  o Women with an unusually short (less than one year) or long (over three years) intervals between pregnancies
  o Women with recurrent miscarriage or stillbirth (three or more miscarriages or still births)
➤ Risk Factors for CP During Pregnancy:
  o Abnormal placental vascular connections (Anastomoses)
  o Twin gestation (C-section prior to onset of labor does not prevent CP in twins)
  o Antepartum hemorrhage (placental separation/abruption)
  o Infection
➤ Risk Factors for CP During Labor/Delivery:
  o Inflammation (infection) of umbilical cord or amniotic membranes
➤ Risk Factors for CP During early postnatal period
  o Low gestational age (prematurity)
  o Acidosis (accumulation of lactic acid in the blood from immature lung system, low Apgar scores, asphyxia (lack of oxygen)
  o Intracranial hemorrhage (IVH)

The four most common conditions found during pregnancies of children who developed cerebral palsy are:
  1. Genetic abnormalities (e.g. birth defects, microcephaly (abnormally small brain), and history of maternal mental retardation)
  2. Birthweight under two thousand grams (2000 g)
  3. Gestational age less than thirty-two weeks
  4. Infection

Office Notes: And into the world came my extremely preterm son.

I'm Sarah, a registered nurse of nearly twenty years, who has worked in ante partum, labor and delivery, post partum and normal newborn nursery, in a small rural Colorado hospital for the past twelve years. I've seen the good and the bad times surrounding birth. I thought tertiary level (usually big city) neonatal intensive care units (NICU) were where a lot of very expensive "experimenting" with very young lives went on. They really shouldn't be keeping the extremely premature alive and the long term quality of life must be poor, were opinions I held.

Those opinions changed!

My pregnancy was cruising along. Very few folks knew I was pregnant, even the folks at the hospital were unaware. Then with a gush my water broke. A tough roller coaster ride began. My predictable life was now not. My opinions of the extreme preterm neonate were in turmoil. What to do?

Off to the hospital I went. Stopping labor progress, with the goal of my transfer to a tertiary hospital, went into full effort. Then via ambulance, leer jet and helicopter, on a snowy April morning, I landed on top of a large city hospital, 180 miles from home.

Then I had two days with a lot of magnesium sulfate running (to stop contractions and buy some time for the baby), and to try to catch my breath. Gee, I'd better think of names, in case this baby comes. Oh, I'd better get the long distance calling card activated. Wow, I can't even lift up the water jug. I was a magnesium noodle!

Then into the world came my baby boy of twenty-six weeks gestation, weighing two pounds and six ounces!

I had a great vaginal delivery, lying on my left side. The room was dimmed, quiet and calm, despite the number of folks. There was my nurse Jenny, delivering doctor, Dr Greg with a great sense of humor, Dr Jan, Neonatologist and two to assist her with Timothy.

I heard Timothy cry and after he was intubated (a tube is placed into the lungs to allow breathing to be assisted) I was able to hold him. He was on a hot pack to keep his temperature up. I looked down in total disbelief to a tiny baby. He was perfect, with a lot of dark hair. Then he was off to the NICU, where he would be for the next three months.

It would be three months of living for the moment, the next phone call or the next visit. Wondering whether the hospital would call with unexpected news of Timothy's deterioration? The unexpected news never came. He did what they expected for a twenty-six week baby. I was lucky!

Reality was hard to grasp. The only way to gain a sense of reality was to look, feel, talk to and hold this baby, my baby. His fragile looking skin made me cautious to touch, his head smaller than my fist and he could not make it around my thumb with his whole hand and fingers. There was no full term "cuddly" baby to hold, but rather a tiny fellow dependent solely on those providing his care. The excitement and joy of a birth was replaced with concern, anxiety and cautious hope.

I returned to work ten days after Timothy's birth. I knew he would have to do his time in the NICU. I had confidence in those caring for him. This was just another day for them. I wanted to be able to have time with him when he did get home, without working as well.

Despite many previous "he might go home" dates, Timothy came home one day shy of his due date, but his coming home was just the beginning…

Office Notes: And into the world came my extremely preterm son, continued...

Early developmental intervention continued with Occupational (OT) and Physical (PT) Therapists coming to our home. Working with games and toys I found many creative ways in our daily life to achieve the therapist's goals. Some ideas the therapists took with them to help others.

I was determined to have Timothy developmentally caught up by the time he started Kindergarten. Every day I tried not to miss an opportunity to help him.

It took a lot of effort. Outsiders saw it as just playing, but it was much more. I knew good long term outcomes were associated highly with the degree of early intervention. You can't start intervention too early, ever!

It may have been three years down the road when I finally took a breath. Timothy's evaluations and follow ups concurred he was caught up to kids of the same age. No more adjusting his age to reflect his prematurity. He was going to be OK. The roller coaster had slowed.

With the roller coaster slowed, I had time to reflect and grieve. No full term pregnancy. I never did feel "really" pregnant. No "cuddly" term baby to hold at birth. No just being Mum and playing with Timothy. Quick there's an OT/PT opportunity, drop the coffee and make it happen. Giving birth to an extremely preterm baby sucks!

Timothy started Kindergarten with no developmental deficit. The effort and work for six years had paid off.

As I look back over the past eight years, I know when you have an extremely preterm baby, very little is the same as the term healthy baby, for Mum or Baby. It's more like a long series of very small stepping stones, some unstable, but which hopefully leads to a great outcome, as is my Timothy.

Chapter 5

Nesting: Twenty-Six to Thirty-Six Weeks

This is one of the best times in pregnancy when all the first and second trimester anxieties have passed, and moms begin to sense fetal movement. Largely due to experiencing fetal movement, the pregnancy goes from being a theoretical event to a tangible being. This chapter covers "the Home Stretch". It addresses normal time frames for delivery and common third trimester symptoms. Birth Plans are treated in detail here and in Chapter Six. Term medical complications and their management are described.

Your Prenatal Visits: Tummy Checks and Heart Tones

Prenatal visits in the third trimester are fairly simple. Your ob provider will ask you about signs and symptoms of preterm labor, high blood pressure, and bleeding problems. They measure the "fundal height". This is the distance between your pubic bone and the top of the uterus. In the third trimester the fundal height in centimeters is equal to the weeks gestation. There can be up to two weeks discrepancy either way. However, more than two weeks will prompt your

> **Third trimester prenatal visits consist of:**
> - **Fundal height**
> - **Fetal heart tones (anything from 120-160 is normal)**
> - **Your weight**
> - **Your blood pressure**
> - **A urine test**

provider to be concerned about excess or insufficient fetal growth and they may order an ultrasound to assess the size of the baby.

These visits will also consist of measuring your weight, blood pressure, listening to the baby's heart rate, and checking urine for protein. These assess your general health and can predict development of gestational diabetes, pre-eclampsia (high blood pressure), and other pregnancy problems.

Ultrasound is not necessary in normal pregnancies. Some of the medical indications for ultrasound in the third trimester are concerns about fetal growth, placental problems, bleeding, and medical illnesses such as diabetes and high blood pressure.

There are only three major lab tests done in the third trimester: screening for gestational diabetes, testing for Rhesus factor and sensitivity, and group B strep screening.

Gestational diabetes: Twenty-Four to Twenty-Eight Weeks

The incidence of gestational diabetes (GD) varies with ethnicity, family history and weight. Some risk factors for gestational diabetes are: history of previous pregnancy with gestational diabetes, history of large babies, family history of diabetes, and certain ethnicities such as Hispanic, African American and Native American.

> **Over half of women with gestational diabetes ultimately develop "adult onset" or "Type II" diabetes later in life.**

You can prevent the onset of gestational diabetes and non-pregnancy related diabetes by managing your diet. Total caloric intake is important as well as intake of refined sugars. Follow the guidelines for weight gain discussed in Chapter One. If you are gaining too much or too little weight, start writing down what you're eating every day. Daily caloric intake for pregnancy is about fourteen calories per pound of body weight, slightly more if you're underweight; slightly less if you're overweight (see BMI table in Chapter One).

Screening for gestational diabetes is done by measuring your blood sugar after a glucose challenge. The glucose challenge can be done with a drink, jelly beans, or a number of other foods, as long as the amount of sugar in the food is a known quantity. Your blood sugar is measured one hour after the glucose challenge. If it exceeds 135 mg/dL you may be asked to do a three hour glucose tolerance test (three-hour GTT). This is the diagnostic test for gestational diabetes. Two abnormal values or a single high fasting value defines gestational diabetes and will prompt treatment.

Many pregnant women have glucose (sugar) in their urine because during pregnancy the kidneys are "leaky"—they cannot filter smaller molecules like glucose so sugar passes into the urine and urine tests are often "positive" for "sugar" at prenatal visits. However, urine tests are not a good way to detect or diagnose diabetes. They are too variable, dependent on time of day, hydration status, and other factors to be reliable.

Most gestational diabetes can be managed with diet. A dietician can instruct you on the principles of a "diabetic diet" and will often give you a specific dietary plan.

Unless it is ignored or inadequately treated gestational diabetes does not usually result in further complications of pregnancy. Its strongest risk is in predicting adult onset diabetes later in life. However you can prevent this through your eating habits and exercise: it is not inevitable.

The most common consequences of GD are big babies, difficult labors, and increased need for Cesarean section, forceps, or vacuum. If your blood sugar is high at the time of delivery the baby can have a rough time with sugar control in the first few days of life. High blood sugars at term also increase the risk of infections. Bacteria feed on sugars so you're at increased risk of uterus infection or wound infection if you have a C-section.

You can prevent most if not all these complications by following your diabetic diet program and controlling weight gain.

Pre-existing diabetes is quite different from gestational diabetes. If you have diabetes prior to becoming pregnant you should definitely consult a health care provider early about pregnancy management. The ideal time is before you even become pregnant. Sugar control in the first trimester is crucial to normal embryonic development.

Pre-eclampsia

Preeclampsia or "toxemia" is a disease of pregnancy defined by high blood pressure and protein in the urine. It affects about ten percent of pregnant women, and usually occurs late in the third trimester. Swelling or "edema" used to be considered part of the diagnosis of pre-eclampsia, however it no longer is. All pregnant women have swelling so it is too non-specific to use to diagnose pre-eclampsia.

If your ob providers suspects you may have pre-eclampsia based on your blood pressure and the presence of protein in your urine, he may order blood tests to evaluate your blood count, kidney, and liver function, as well as an ultrasound or other test to evaluate the fetal well-being.

The exact cause of pre-eclampsia is not known but it is thought to be related to a factor made by the placenta, as it resolves after delivery of the baby and placenta. It is also believed to have something to do with the immune system. Pregnancy by a new father can cause pre-eclampsia in someone who did not have it in a prior pregnancy. Oddly, women who engage in oral sex have a lower incidence of pre-eclampsia.

Some of the most prominent risk factors for pre-eclampsia include age over thirty-five or under fifteen; prior history of high blood pressure or pre-eclampsia; and being overweight.

There is some evidence that calcium supplementation at the level of two thousand (2000) mg daily can prevent pre-eclampsia in people who've had it before, are in their first pregnancy, or have high blood pressure preceding pregnancy.

Pre-eclampsia usually resolves with delivery. However, if you're remote from delivery your ob provider may put you to bed rest. At term, more severe forms of pre-eclampsia are treated with delivery and magnesium sulfate. Magnesium sulfate prevents **eclampsia**, the onset of seizures related to high blood pressures and other changes of pre-eclampsia. Magnesium sulfate also lowers maternal blood pressure. Once you've delivered usually the magnesium sulfate is discontinued about twenty-four hours post delivery because by this time the danger period is resolved.

Rhesus Factor (Rh Factor): Twenty-Six to Twenty-Eight weeks

Another blood test done in the third trimester, often with the diabetes test, is screening for Rhesus factor and "sensitization" to Rhesus factor. Rhesus factor is a protein on blood cells. When your blood type is described as (A, B, or O) positive, it means you carry the Rhesus factor. If you're Rh positive you have no further worries and can move on.

Up to thirteen percent of people are negative for the Rhesus factor, depending on ethnicity. If you're negative for the Rhesus factor (e.g. "type (A, B, or O-negative blood") this means your red blood cells do not have the rhesus protein on their surfaces. This is of little consequence to you but can be of serious consequences if your baby is Rh-positive and you've become

Common Causes of Rh Sensitization
- **Cordocentesis (amniocentesis to obtain a sample of fetal cord blood)** 30-50%
- **Miscarriage** 3-5%
- **Elective pregnancy termination** 6-20%
- **Ectopic pregnancy** 5-8%
- **Amniocentesis** 4-11%
- **Chorionic Villus Sampling** 8-15%

"sensitized" to the Rhesus factor. It is unusual to become sensitized to the Rhesus factor. It can only occur if there is significant exposure of fetal blood to your blood. In this event, you can develop antibodies, immune proteins, against Rhesus factor. These antibodies do not usually affect the pregnancy in which you're sensitized because they are synthesized at low levels. However, they can affect future pregnancies.

Most people who become Rhesus sensitized are not aware they're sensitized, nor do they remember when they became sensitized. Sensitization can occur with miscarriage or with unperceived passage of blood from the fetal system to the maternal system. The latter would require some type of breakdown in the placental barrier, which is rare.

If you're Rh negative you'll often receive "Rhogam" as a precaution against sensitization. Rhogam binds up any Rhesus proteins in your circulation and prevents you from becoming sensitized. Rhogam is given any time there is a risk of maternal exposure to fetal cells, such as with a miscarriage, amniocentesis, or placental hemorrhage. Rhogam is also often given routinely at twenty-six to twenty-eight weeks if you're Rh negative. You won't necessarily be tested for sensitization prior to receiving Rhogam because it's usually cheaper to give the immunization, rather than test for sensitization prior to immunization.

Group B Strep Culture (Thirty-Six to Thirty-Seven weeks)

Group B strep is a bacterium that can live in the genital tract of up to fifteen percent of women. Group B strep can come and go—you can carry it for a few weeks, get rid of it, and then carry it again later. Group B strep does not usually cause symptoms in women. However, sometimes it can lead to vaginal infection, especially if your immune system is suppressed by stress or a medical illness such as diabetes.

Group B strep can cause pneumonia and severe infection in newborns because they have not developed immunity to it before birth. Babies can only become exposed to Group B Strep in labor once the water has broken.

Group B strep (GBS) vaginal culture is done close to term to determine if you're a carrier of the bacteria at time of delivery. If you're GBS positive you will be given antibiotics during labor to prevent the baby from contracting GBS.

Physical Changes in the Third Trimester

The baby grows, you retain more fluid; and this magnifies physical symptoms.

Pelvic Pressure

As the baby grows to occupy a greater portion of the uterus, relative to the fluid volume and placenta, pelvic pressure increases. The presenting part (most downward part) of the baby puts more pressure on the pelvic muscles, the lower back, the bones, and joints. This causes sciatica (nerve pain that shoots down the back of the leg), pubic symphysis pain (pain in the front of the pelvis), pelvic pressure, and urinary frequency. These symptoms can change as the baby shifts position, rotates, and moves.

Warm baths, cat stretches and some yoga positions relieve pelvic pressure, sciatica, and back pain. Sometimes changing your position can make the baby move enough to alleviate pressure on a given area.

A heating pad (on a low setting) and acetaminophen (Tylenol) can relieve pubic bone pain.

Constipation

The pregnancy hormone, progesterone, slows intestinal movement and can increase constipation. It is important to drink a lot of fluid and exercise regularly to minimize constipation. Walking is great for improvement of bowel motility. Certain foods such as peanut butter and cheese, anything with lots of saturated fats, can be particularly constipating during pregnancy.

Sleep Changes

Insomnia can become more predominant in the third trimester. Many factors cause pregnancy insomnia: frequent trips to the bathroom at night, physical discomfort, anticipation of the new baby, and anxiety about the new baby. Many people have vivid dreams during the third trimester. Some of these dreams are catastrophic, "worst case scenario" visions. These are usually triggered by ill-defined fear of the unknown. All these questions flood in: Will my baby be normal? Will I be a good parent? How will this affect our relationship? Can I count on my partner to be a good parent?

These fears go both ways: Potential mothers and fathers all experience them to some degree.

Many over-the-counter sleep aids are effective and safe for pregnancy insomnia. However, if you have severe insomnia with multiple sequential nights of inadequate sleep, consult your ob provider for possible additional treatment.

Braxton Hicks Contractions

Braxton Hicks contractions (BHC's) increase in the third trimester. It is not unusual to have "runs" of BHC's—say ten in an hour followed by none. BHC's frequently occur in the evening hours between six PM and midnight. As long as they subside within an hour or two of rest and fluid, these are not preterm labor contractions.

Breast Leakage

By twenty weeks your milk-producing hormones increase. You may notice breast leakage as early as the late first trimester, especially if you've breast-fed in the past. Intercourse, breast manipulation, and a crying baby can bring on breast leakage.

Nesting

Nesting is the urge to clean house and prepare for the baby. Most women experience a few weeks of nesting at some point in the third trimester. Some people are tempted to overdo it and do something like a major remodel. It is wise to resist this temptation. Overexertion and exhaustion can lead to preterm labor, blood pressure problems, and other pregnancy complications.

Vaginal Discharge

Many people get a white or mucusy discharge in the third trimester. The mucus plug is a collection of mucus that fills the cervical canal. It is made by glands in the cervix. The mucus plug is constantly "turning over"—being replaced as old mucus sloughs off and new mucus is formed. You can "lose your mucus plug" a month or six weeks before you actually go into labor. Sometimes the mucus plug is accompanied by old brown blood.

White discharge is due to rapid production and sloughing of vaginal cells related to estrogen and progesterone. It is "physiologic" or normal as long as it doesn't have an odor and is not irritating.

Sex in the Third Trimester

Sex in the third trimester is interesting. As the baby descends or settles into the pelvis you and your partner may feel more "pressure" or other sensations with intercourse. Your partner may feel like he's "bumping into" the baby. He might be, but this does not cause any problems. He cannot "hurt" the baby. Intercourse is not associated with preterm labor. However, intercourse can sometimes stimulate a short bout of contractions. These usually subside within an hour.

Intercourse is safe as long as it's not associated with sustained hours of contractions or vaginal bleeding.

Emotional Status

Late in the third trimester, many hormone levels are "out of sight". High hormone levels can lead to unpredictable mood swings: ecstatic one minute, crying the next. There may be no rhyme or reason to these emotional changes.

Some people experience depression in the third trimester, or even earlier. If you're feeling overwhelmed or in "funk" you just can't seem to shake off, you may be depressed and you should consult your ob provider.

Progesterone relieves anxiety. It reaches very high levels in the third trimester. However, as you approach labor, and after delivery progesterone and estrogen drop precipitously. This may trigger anxiety, baby blues, or depression.

Negative emotions respond to a brisk walk, relaxation exercises, and deep breathing. However, in serious situations with intractable sadness, you may need to use an anti-depressant. Most anti-depressant medications are safe in pregnancy. If you have depression prior to pregnancy or if depression and anxiety run in your family you are more prone to these conditions and you should have a low threshold for asking your health care provider if your symptoms could be related to depression or anxiety.

Normal Fetal Movement and Sleep Cycles; Fetal Breathing

Fetal movement slows down in the third trimester. The baby occupies more and more space in the uterus, and simply doesn't have as much freedom of motion as in early pregnancy. Third tri-

> **Fetal "nap" sessions can last up to two hours and are normal periods of inactivity.**

mester fetuses often act like newborns and take "naps". These are termed "sleep cycles". A sleep cycle may last about two hours. During a sleep cycle you won't feel the baby move much if at all. Then it can "wake up", move quite a bit, and enter another sleep cycle.

At minimum you should feel the baby make at least ten movements in a two hour period. These may not be large movements—they may just be "twitches" of a limb. Most people feel fetal move-

> **Fetal "breathing" occurs intermittently and is brief, lasting seconds or minutes.**

ment in the evenings when they are resting and can pay attention to the baby. When you're busy during the day you may not feel the baby moving at all. The baby actually is moving but your own activity can mask the perception of fetal movement.

Hiccoughs ("hiccups") are normal and feel like a rhythmic "thumping" or twitching of the baby. Usually hiccoughs are episodic and last a few minutes, but sometimes they persist for hours. Hiccoughs are a normal process of the maturation of the diaphragm (breathing) muscle.

After twenty weeks gestation the fetus can also be seen on ultrasound to exhibit "breathing" motion. This is a rapid expansion/contraction of the chest and is thought to be part of the process of maturing the rib and breathing muscles in preparation for life outside the womb. Fetal breathing is brief—often lasting no more than thirty seconds to two minutes. Fetuses may have bouts of "breathing" every few minutes or once every half-hour to hour, depending on how active the baby is at the time.

Prenatal Classes

People usually begin prenatal classes after thirty weeks gestation. The closer to delivery you begin your prenatal classes, the more likely you are to retain the information. Everyone has a different opinion and a different birth story so take the stories you hear in prenatal classes as just that: your experience will be unique, unlike anyone else's.

Most prenatal classes review the basics of labor, different breathing techniques, and medical interventions.

Perineal Massage

Perineal massage has become talked about as a way to prevent or minimize vaginal tears. The best way to minimize vaginal tears is to control delivery of the head (see pictures in labor chapter).

Perineal massage involves using the thumb and forefingers to massage the vaginal opening with the idea of preventing tears during delivery. Massage oil is essential or it can be uncomfortable. There is no scientific evidence supporting perineal massage as a way to reduce tears.

What to pack

Much of what you may deem essential, actually isn't. The only thing you really need to take the baby home from the hospital is a car seat. Some hospitals will check your car seat before you are discharged, to make sure the baby is well supported, and you are familiar with its use. However, here is a packing list for things that might be useful.

Hold off on purchasing lactation bras until your milk comes in as your breast size may change substantially when it does come in.

Birth Plans

Chapter Six on Labor addresses birth plans in detail. Although you should be thinking about specifics you'd like to see happen during your birth, keep in mind labor can be unpredictable. The goal is a healthy baby and a healthy mom. If not everything goes "according to plan", rejoice in the fact you have a healthy baby and don't sweat the small stuff.

Essential
- Clothes for labor that can get messy and be thrown away if necessary
- Car Seat
- Diapers

Useful
- Baby blankets, outfits, and "onesies"
- Double Electric Breast Pump

Would be nice
- Camera
- Music

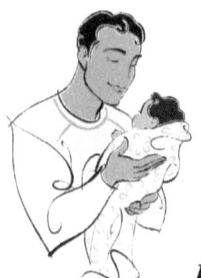

For Dads: Pregnancy "Mania"

Don't be surprised if at times your wife is running around the house in a seemingly non-stop frenzy; while at other times she's collapsed asleep on the couch or may be in tears. The frenetic preparations can both be a relief for stress and a cause for stress. Your wife may appear to be compulsive about things you just don't consider important.

If your wife is running around frantically preparing for things, ask her what you can do to help. When she spouts out a mother-of-all to-do list that could suck up years of your life, ask her to prioritize—what needs to be done now, what can wait, and what can simply be forever ignored. Many of the things on our to-do list are not as important as we think they are; and if we give it time, the imperativeness of this or that item may evaporate.

Don't be too insistent about revising the "to-do" list—this may only get you into trouble. Often the best option is to start in on the to-do list and help out.

Chapter 6

It's Time! Labor and Delivery Me

The only thing predictable about labor and delivery is it is not. You can't foresee or control it. This is a law of nature. Don't fight it, or it will best you.

> **Condition your body and your mind for labor.**

Keys to Successful Vaginal Birth: **P**assenger, **P**elvis, **P**ower

The keys to delivering vaginally without assistance lie with the size and position of the baby (passenger), the size and shape of your pelvis, and the power of the uterine contractions. Any of the following factors can impact whether you need assistance: if the baby is too large, or in a poor position to deliver; if your pelvis is narrow or oddly shaped; or if the uterus doesn't produce enough force with contractions, or loses strength during labor.

You have some control over these things. For example, if you control your weight you are more likely to have an "average" size baby that can fit through the pelvis. You're less likely to develop medical illness during pregnancy such as diabetes, high blood pressure, and pre-eclampsia. A huge body of evidence has amassed to show excess weight and obesity increase the C-section rate.

Condition Your Body for Labor: You Can Affect the Outcome

If you maintain good physical condition during pregnancy your likely to have better "power" come time to deliver. For one, you will be stronger; you'll have greater stamina and better muscle tone. You'll be more effective with pushing. All these factors lower your risk and improve your odds of a safe vaginal delivery without medical intervention.

A good exercise during pregnancy is walking thirty to sixty minutes daily. You can do almost any exercise during pregnancy, including lifting weights, if you do it sensibly. Use good body mechanics with weights—lift with your legs, not your back. Don't overdo it. Small dumbbells (two, three, and five pound) are safe to use because they won't throw you off balance, and you'll be less tempted to over exert yourself.

With any exercise, make sure you keep your heart rate under 140 beats per minute. You can calculate your heart rate by timing your pulse for six seconds and multiplying by ten.

Condition Your Mind: Abdominal Breathing and Progressive Muscle Relaxation

During pregnancy and labor we have a tendency to hyperventilate. This means we breathe shallow and fast from our chest up, instead of using our abdominal muscles to breathe. The hormone, progesterone, can make you feel "out of breath". Moreover, the baby displaces your lungs upward and actually decreases the volume of air you can take with each breath. This physical state of hyperventilation can make you feel emotional, anxious, have numb hands and feet, and increase the tendency to "worry". Slow deep breaths relieve hyperventilation, and subsequently improve anxiety.

Our physical state can affect our frame of mind. If you are constantly rushing and fail to breathe deeply you can create a state of anxiety within yourself simply by being physically "uptight".

Try this for one minute per day throughout your pregnancy: Whatever you're doing stop for one minute and practice **abdominal breathing**. Fill the bases of your lungs by visualizing your diaphragm muscles pushing downward so your abdomen pushes outward with inhalation. Exhale slowly. Do this for five breaths. Do not rush.

Progressive muscle relaxation is a great technique for calming yourself if you're feeling particularly emotional or anxious. Get comfortable lying down or reclining in a chair. Put on some soothing music. Take a deep breath in and clench your fists as hard as you can for five to ten seconds. Let them relax for twenty seconds, then move on to your biceps. Do this with all the major muscle groups in your body in the following sequence:

Fists
Biceps (front upper arm muscles)
Triceps (back upper arm muscles)
Face (scrunch it up)
Jaw (open it wide)
Neck (scrunch it up)
Shoulders (scrunch)
Buttocks

Quadriceps (front upper leg muscles)
Hamstrings (back upper leg muscles)
Calves (point your toes)
Shin muscles (flex your ankles)

Your Birth Plan

You have a lot of control to enhance your labor and improve your delivery experience. We see many similar requests in birth plans. Most people want as minimal intervention as possible. They want their baby on the tummy, for dad to cut the cord; and to be able to breast-feed right away. If you're going to develop a birth plan discuss it with your ob provider in the last month of pregnancy, before you actually arrive in labor. If you address it ahead of time questions can be answered and you're more likely to make your provider aware of your wishes and align her behavior with your goals. Ob providers and labor nurses want you and your family to be happy, and to have a good birth experience.

If you want special music, bring it. Lighting can be adjusted by you or the labor staff.

There are some things to be aware of regarding birth plans. You, the labor nurses, and the ob provider are to a large extent "at the mercy" of your labor. There are some things you and they can affect, and others that are completely out of their and your hands.

If you have high expectations or rigid ideas about how you will deliver you can be disappointed in direct proportion to your expectations. It seems to me, after years of delivering babies, people with detailed prescriptions about how things will go, often have more difficult labors and are more likely to wind up with a Cesarean section or difficult birth, than families who approach labor with a relaxed but positive attitude and are willing to make adjustments in their expectations. If you're the type of person who writes a ten-page single-spaced birth plan, highlighted in red, underlined and bolded (yes, I have seen these), caution: you may be disappointed. There's an unofficial rule well known to labor nurses and ob providers that the likelihood of a C-section is directly proportional to the length and detail of the woman's "birth plan".

You probably would like to know when It will happen, how long It will take, and whether or not you really will need pain medicine. Here are the definitive answers to these questions: It won't

> **Expectations: Make your life easy and keep it simple.**

happen soon enough *or* it will happen before you're ready. It will take way too long or will be much faster than you thought; and it will hurt less or more than you expect.

Some labors will be quick and uneventful, while others may take days and require medical intervention to accomplish the deed. Cheekiness aside, read on for some real answers to these and other questions.

When Will it Happen?

The average length of gestation in the United States is 282 days (forty weeks and two days from the first date of the last menstrual period). This takes into account both spontaneous and induced labor. Remember—a due date is more like a "due month" and you can safely deliver anywhere from thirty-seven weeks onward. A mere five percent of women actually deliver *on* their due date, and some of these are induced. If you go past your due date most ob providers induce labor around or before forty-two weeks gestation, depending on your specific circumstances.

Exact due dates really only come into play if your ob provider is considering inducing your labor for one reason or another and is trying to establish whether the baby has matured enough to induce labor.

Your ob provider may have revised your due date if you weren't sure of your last menstrual period and an ultrasound showed a due date significantly different from that given by your last menstrual period. If you're confused about your due date ask your ob provider if it was revised by ultrasound or to clarify any discrepancies between your menstrual dates and ultrasound dating.

If there is a question as to whether your baby is mature enough to be delivered, and you need to be induced for some reason, the ob provider may perform an amniocentesis to determine lung maturity. This is rare (less than one percent of pregnancies) and usually only occurs if prenatal care started too late to obtain good dating information; or if you are preterm and need to be delivered for a medical reason.

How Long Will it Take?

The length of labor depends on how you define the start of labor. Ninety-five percent of women admitted to the hospital for spontaneous labor will deliver within ten hours of arrival. The average

> **True Labor = Regular Contractions + Cervical Dilation**

time for first labors is about ten hours, and for subsequent labors, is about six hours. This definition considers the beginning of **true labor** to be **the onset of**

regular uterine contractions accompanied by dilation of the cervix. Much can happen before true labor begins and contractions can start days, weeks, or months before the onset of true labor.

Phases of labor

Early labor can last up to twenty hours and is the gradual onset of contractions which result in softening and thinning of the cervix, but without much cervical dilation. Prior to her first labor, a woman begins labor with a cervix that is long, thick and closed. This means the cervix is about two inches long, is positioned at the back of the vagina behind the fetal head, and is firm to touch. Throughout labor, contractions soften the cervix, thin (efface) it completely, and open it (dilate) to about ten centimeters to allow the fetal head to move down the birth canal. **Early labor** can take anywhere from a few hours to a day and produces gradual changes in the cervix from long, thick and closed to mostly thinned out, softer, and dilated anywhere from one to three centimeters.

Active labor occurs with the onset of regular contractions every few minutes accompanied by further dilation and effacement of the cervix. Most women are considered to be in active labor by the time they reach three centimeters dilation. However some women who have had previous labors can actually begin to dilate painlessly in the latter half of the third trimester. Occasionally women who have had prior babies will be three or more centimeters dilated before true labor even begins.

Cervical effacement and dilation make up the **first stage of labor**. The first stage encompasses early and active labor, and the fetal head gradually moves down the birth canal. This is called

> **First Stage = Onset of regular contractions to complete cervical dilation.**

descent. The first stage of labor averages nine hours in a woman who hasn't had a baby before, and five hours in women who have had prior babies. Once the cervix is fully dilated, you'll enter the second stage of labor and begin pushing.

The **second stage of labor** is the time between complete cervical dilation and delivery of the infant. During second stage the baby moves down and out of the birth canal with the help of the mother pushing. The length of the second stage of labor is to some degree dependent on your pushing efforts and averages one hour if it's your first baby and you

> **Second stage = Complete cervical dilation to delivery of the baby.**

don't have an epidural, to twenty minutes if you've had a previous baby. It is not uncommon for the second stage of labor to take two or three hours and sometimes require assistance from your ob provider. The length of second stage is affected by your pushing force, the shape of your pelvis, the size and position of the baby, and other anatomic factors, such as if you're overweight.

The **third stage of labor** is the delivery of the placenta and can take anywhere from a few minutes to half an hour. Usually your ob provider will have you push a little to deliver the placenta.

> **Third Stage = Delivery of infant to delivery of placenta.**

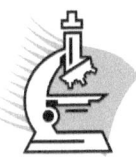

Science Notes: What causes labor to begin?

Despite the fact billions of babies have been born on the planet, no one knows exactly how human labor begins.

In non-primate mammals such as sheep, there is good evidence that labor is initiated by both progesterone withdrawal (a drop in progesterone levels), and by signals from the fetus. The fetal sheep seems to send out a chemical message it is mature. These impulses are thought to be produced by the fetal sheep adrenal glands.

In humans, however, labor is not initiated by progesterone withdrawal; and although it's a neat theory to imagine the mature fetus sends a signal for labor to begin, there is no scientific evidence to support this. We do know certain hormones and chemicals are important in the second and third stage of labor.

Oxytocin

Oxytocin is a hormone produced by the pituitary gland located in the brain. Oxytocin stimulates uterine contractions and is important in sustaining labor. However, labor is not preceded by dramatic increases in oxytocin concentration in the blood stream. Oxytocin levels rise throughout labor and are highest during advanced cervical dilation, then delivery of the baby and placenta. Oxytocin is also crucial to initiation of lactation and to the milk "let down" response. It stimulates small muscles around the milk ducts to eject milk from the breast.

Although we know onset of labor is not preceded by a dramatic increase in oxytocin levels, we do know that labor can be induced (started artificially) with a synthetic version of oxytocin called pitocin.

Pressure of the baby's head on the cervix can also stimulate release of oxytocin and prostaglandins (see below).

Prostaglandins

Prostaglandins are hormones produced by the fetus and the uterine lining, the decidua, in pregnancy. (The non-pregnant uterine lining is called the endometrium—this is what you shed every month when you have a period.)

Prostaglandins are elevated throughout labor. Although they are produced by the baby and the uterine lining, there is no evidence that a dramatic increase in prostaglandins from these sources initiates labor.

Prostaglandins have two major effects: 1) Soften and shorten the cervix. 2) Produce uterine contractions.

Although we know prostaglandins are not solely responsible for initiating labor, they can be used, like pitocin to induce labor. Artificial prostaglandins come in pills (Cytotec, misoprostol), gels (Cervidil, Prepidil). If prostaglandins are used to induce labor, it is usually in the setting of a cervix that is "long, thick, and closed" and has not undergone much softening, effacement (thinning), or dilation.

There are many other chemicals and hormones involved in the initiation and maintenance of labor but the exact mechanism by which onset of labor transpires remains a mystery.

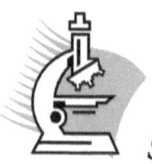

Science Notes: What causes labor to begin?
(Continued)

Changes in uterine muscle

Before and during labor, uterine muscle cells undergo two major transformations. The first is the formation of cell-to-cell communication channels called "gap junctions". Gap junctions allow individual uterine muscle cells to "talk" to each other through chemical transmission and provide for the synchronized action of many muscles cells to cause a coordinated uterine contraction.

Uterine muscles cells also change in their receptor status. They develop an increased number of receptors for oxytocin, prostaglandins, and other chemicals important to the initiation of labor.

Changes in the baby

Prior to labor the baby's movement may slow down. This is normal as long as the baby is moving at least ten times in a two hour period while you're paying attention. When labor begins the baby's spine extends slightly from the curled position, and the baby may gain as much as five to ten centimeters in elongation as labor progresses. More on this later …

Early, prodromal, and false labor

Early, prodromal, and false labor can be difficult to distinguish from one another. **Early labor** can consist of regular or somewhat irregular contractions that do soften, shorten, *and dilate* the cervix. **Prodromal labor** is regular or irregular contractions that do not produce cervical dilation, but can produce some softening and effacement. However, prodromal labor usually occurs at thirty-nine weeks or greater in gestation. It sometimes lasts for days and can evolve into true early labor.

False labor consists of regular uterine contractions that do not produce any cervical change. False labor can occur anywhere from thirty-seven weeks onward and sometimes persists for weeks. False labor can be intermittent; and can last for hours or days. It can mimic prodromal labor and early labor.

> **False Labor = Contractions without cervical change. It can mimic true labor and be distinguished only by examining the cervix.**

It can even be painful enough to require pain medication. However, false labor is defined by absence of cervical change.

False labor and prodromal labor can result in admission to the hospital for several reasons. One is to observe the labor pattern to define whether it's false labor, prodromal labor, or true early labor. A second reason can be to administer pain medication or sedation (to induce sleep). False labor can be very frustrating because it is uterine contractions that can be persistent, exhausting, or painful. Sedation with pain medication will usually eradicate false labor or prodromal labor, thus distinguishing these from true labor, and providing relief from pain and exhaustion. True labor will not be arrested by the sedation or pain medication used to manage false labor.

Spontaneous rupture of the membranes (breaking the water)

Spontaneous rupture of the membranes or breaking your water usually occurs during early or active labor. However ten percent of women experience rupture of the membranes before labor begins. At term this is called "pre-

> **Liquefaction of the cervical mucus and leaking urine is often confused with leaking amniotic fluid.**

mature rupture of the membranes" because it occurs before the onset of contractions. This is not to be confused with "preterm rupture of the membranes" in which the bag of water breaks before thirty-seven weeks gestation (see Chapter Five).

If your water breaks it is unmistakable. You may wake up in a pool of fluid on the bed, or it may soak through your clothes if you're up and about. When the water breaks, it is often a large volume, although rarely a woman will leak fluid. Rupture of the amniotic fluid typically produces constant uncontrollable watery vaginal seepage or discharge. Sometimes people confuse liquefaction of the cervical mucus plug or leakage of urine with rupture of the membranes. These are different and can be distinguished by a cervical exam, possibly in conjunction with ultrasound to assess the amniotic fluid volume, if there's any question.

If your water breaks before the onset of labor, contractions ensue spontaneously most of the time. However, if contractions don't begin within a certain time frame (six to twelve hours) your ob provider may induce labor to prevent your bag of waters from being ruptured for so long it increases the risk of infection to you and your baby. The risk of infection increases substantially if the bag of waters has been ruptured for eighteen hours or more and you haven't yet delivered.

Usually the amniotic fluid is "clear" or straw colored. It may contain flecks of white material in it called **vernix**. This is a protective waxy substance that coats the baby's skin so the baby doesn't get "water logged" or "prune skin". Occasionally the amniotic fluid is green tinged or bloody. Green tinge is called meconium staining and it means the baby has had a bowel movement *in utero*. Bloody fluid often results simply from cervical dilation; but it can be the sign of something more severe. Notify your ob provider or go to the hospital if your water breaks or if you have bright red vaginal bleeding like a menstrual period.

Bloody show

Labor and bleeding go hand in hand. Consider labor the most colossal menstrual period of your life and you won't be disappointed. However, instead of a few days of cramps you get major pains, possibly hemorrhoids, and a baby out of it.

> **Active labor and bleeding go hand-in-hand—due to cervical dilation.**

Bleeding at the *onset* of labor is most commonly caused by passage of the mucus plug (usually old brown blood with mucus). Bleeding *during* labor is most likely due to dilation of the cervix, and bleeding at the *end* of labor occurs with vaginal tearing and passage of the placenta. Rarely bleeding can signify something more serious, especially after twenty weeks and you should notify your ob provider or go to the hospital for sustained bright red bleeding.

The Delivery Center

Much of the anxiety surrounding labor results not only from the thought of pain and fear of the unknown, but also what the delivery center will be like. Who will attend the birth—someone I know and like or someone I don't know well or care for much? What will my labor nurse be like? Some of this may be alleviated with a tour of labor and delivery at some point during your third trimester. A tour is often a component of prenatal classes.

The Labor Nurse

Most people don't realize your labor nurse will spend a lot more time with you during the birth of your baby than will your ob provider, be they midwife or doctor. Labors can last hours, some-

> **Your labor nurse will by your most consistent companion.**

times days. Most midwives and doctors have offices to run, other patients to see, and a family to attend to if it's after regular business hours. Your labor nurse is a very important part of your birth experience.

Unless there is a problem the doctor or midwife may see you occasionally during the early parts of labor, but won't be called to the bedside by your labor nurse until you're in advanced cervical dilation or are ready to push.

Labor nurses are trained to support and coach women through all aspects of labor, including breathing techniques, positioning during labor, pain management, pushing, and initiation of breast-feeding. I encourage you to establish a good rapport with your labor nurse by showing her respect for her knowledge and experience. Although they don't have the "M.D.", "D.O.", or "C.N.M." behind their name, some labor nurses have more experience with birth than the midwife or doctor who will deliver your baby. This doesn't mean the nurse should do your delivery—she has neither the licensing nor the liability coverage to do so. However, recognize your nurse can be a tremendous asset to your birth experience.

Your labor nurse always wishes you to have a good birth experience—that is their job. As with any profession, medicine included, you will have more confidence in some of your nurses and less in others. Some of that may relate to their perceived age or experience level, or just personal chemistry. If you find you are having so much friction with a labor nurse you feel it's affecting your birth experience there is usually a supervisor present who can address major incompatibilities. Sometimes, if you give people the benefit of the doubt, what started off as a rocky relationship may prove to be a wonderful and supportive one.

Labor nurses work in shifts, so you may have one, two, three or more nurses throughout your labor, especially if your labor lasts longer than average. Remember, averages are computed from a pool of people, about half of whom have shorter labors, and half have longer labors. Thus, you have roughly a fifty percent chance of having a longer labor than "average".

When the baby is crowning, or just about ready to come, your labor nurse will usually call for a "baby nurse". A second nurse will arrive to assist with the baby so your labor nurse can focus on your medical needs.

Other non-Ob-Provider Delivery Personnel

Baby Care Providers

Your delivery may be attended by a pediatrician or neonatal nurse practitioner (NNP) if called for by your ob provider. Most ob providers will call for a pediatrician or NNP to attend the birth if they feel the baby may need extra attention after birth. It is routine to request a pediatrician or NNP if you have an operative vaginal delivery (vacuum or forceps) or a C-section.

Nursing and Medical Students

If you deliver at a hospital that trains medical or nursing students, your birth may be observed or attended by a student. Usually your permission is sought beforehand and the student appears at the time of delivery. Sometimes the student will also be available to support you in labor.

At teaching universities, medical students or midwifery students will sometimes perform the delivery under the immediate supervision of a teaching medical resident or midwife. Delivery under these circumstances is as safe as delivery by a midwife or physician who has completed training. There is usually a system of successively more experienced personnel available from residents up to senior physicians and midwives, should complications arise.

The Labor Room or LDR

Fathers no longer pace anxiously in sterile waiting rooms, waiting to learn the news and pass out the cigars. Gone are the days when a woman labored in a gurney in a vomit-green tiled room and was transported to a delivery room/operating room for the birth. Welcome to the LDR!

Now is the best time in history to have a baby in the developed world. Mortality rates of mothers and term infants are near zero. The hospital "Maternity Ward" has evolved into the "Family Birth Place". The homey LDR (Labor, Delivery, and Recovery Room) has replaced the sterile "closet" tiled in puce where women labored on gurneys and were transported to an operating room for delivery. Now women labor in rooms decorated like family bedrooms, complete with faux-wood flooring, curtains, real furniture such as rocking chairs, a bed for dad; jetted hot tubs and private bathrooms with large showers. Much of the medical equipment is discreetly hidden in cabinets so as to make the process of birth feel as natural as possible. It appears at essential moments so as to minimize its intrusiveness. The only medical equipment immediately visible is the fetal monitor and the infant warmer.

The gurney has been replaced by the labor bed which can support a woman in any position: lying, seated, or squatting. The bottom of the bed can be removed to access "stirrups" (now more like foot rests) should the mother desire to use them for leverage and balance during pushing. The labor bed also allows access for your ob provider. You will generally remain in your LDR, or at least call it home base, for the duration of your labor and delivery.

A paradigm shift has occurred in the mentalities and orientation of obstetric care providers and labor nurses. The paternalistic doctor-patient or nurse-patient model has been abandoned and providers now view themselves as expert support personnel. They see their role as imperative to create as safe, individualized and fulfilling a birth experience as possible for everyone who walks through their doors. Women and families are much more empowered in their birth experience than they were fifty or even twenty years ago. They possess more information about their options and are savvier.

Depending on the hospital, there is much flexibility on who's allowed to attend the birth. Of course the baby's father or your significant support person may be present. But in some places you may be allowed to have your parents, your other children, your siblings, in-laws, Uncle Joe and Great Grandpa Henry attend your birth as well (if you like). During actual delivery of the infant, most places will "shoo" everyone out of the room except for one or two crucial support people out of necessity for your and the baby's safety. Emergencies may arise which necessitate calling in extra hospital personnel. At this point the room can become awfully crowded, and to allow the hospital personnel to maneuver about the room and do their jobs, your relatives may be shown to the waiting area.

The Fetal Monitor

Every modern labor room is equipped with a **cardiotocodynamometer**. This is a machine with two sensors: one to

> **There is no specific fetal heart rate pattern during labor that predicts cerebral palsy.**

determine pressure from uterine contractions (the "**tocodynamometer**"); and a Doppler to measure the fetal heart rate (the "**cardio**"). These values can be obtained by external monitors placed on the maternal abdomen, or by internal monitors. Internal monitors will be discussed in detail later.

Over the past forty years electronic fetal monitoring has become the standard of care for labor in the United States. There are two approaches to fetal monitoring: Continuous electronic fetal monitoring and intermittent auscultation. The former is what it says: continuous. The latter is listening to the fetal heart rate at fifteen-to thirty-minute intervals during early labor, five-minute intervals during active labor, and with contractions during pushing.

Continuous electronic fetal monitoring has generated controversy in recent years because it's become entrenched in our current system of labor management, without having been demonstrated to be of clear benefit over intermittent auscultation. Make no mistake: Monitoring of the fetus during labor *does* save fetal and maternal lives. However, during the past forty years, research has shown no reduction in intrapartum fetal death or cerebral palsy rates with continuous fetal monitoring versus intermittent auscultation.

The Fetal Heart Rate During Labor

The fetal heart rate is described as having a "baseline" which is usually between 120 and 160 beats per minute. It is not unusual, nor does it necessarily cause stress to the baby for the baseline to drop below 120 or go above 160 from time to time during labor. The fetal heart rate is not monotonous. From time to time, especially with fetal movement, the heart rate "accelerates" or

> **Continuous electronic fetal heart rate monitoring has not reduced the incidence of cerebral palsy over the past fifty years. In fact, the incidence has increased, in large part due to the survival of extremely premature infants.**

increases fifteen or more beats above the baseline for fifteen seconds. Similarly, the fetal heart rate can drop below the baseline. Mild drops in the fetal heart rate, such as to ninety beats per minute do not cause the baby any lasting ill effects. Even severe brief (less than two minute) drops, such as to sixty beats per minute do not cause the baby adverse effects, as long as these are not persistent or repetitive. Research has shown a low heart rate such as sixty beats per minute must be sustained for a period of time such as ten minutes or greater to cause ill effects to the baby. Even so, these ill effects are often self-limited and result in no persistent problems.

Multiple factors can affect the fetal heart rate when the uterus contracts during labor. The compression forces of the uterine muscle can alter the blood supply to the placenta, sometimes producing a drop in fetal heart rate. These same forces can exert pressure on the umbilical cord resulting in drops in the fetal heart rate. Moreover, the pressure of the

> **The healthy fetal heart rate varies from 120 to 160 beats per minute. However, brief segments outside this range are normal and result in no permanent ill effects.**

fetal head against the cervix can cause slight declines in the fetal heart rate baseline. Most of these decreases in the fetal heart rate are brief and inconsequential to the fetal oxygenation status. These changes do not result in cerebral palsy, mental retardation, or fetal demise. The baby is very resilient and can sustain even severe drops in fetal heart rate.

Maternal Position Change and Administration of Oxygen by Mask

It is best to allow the baby to "recover" from brief drops in the heart rate *in utero*, without medical intervention. Changes in maternal position facilitate uterine blood flow and recovery of the fetal heart rate to baseline. Moreover, administration of oxygen to the mother may increase the level of oxygen in the maternal bloodstream. Such an increase could be transmitted through the placenta to improve the baby's oxygenation status during labor. The placenta does an excellent job of nourishing the baby throughout labor and can act as a buffer between changes in maternal status, contractions, and the baby's response to these changes in heart rate.

Cerebral Palsy and Intrapartum Hypoxia

Research has shown that over ninety-five percent of cerebral palsy is caused by an event during pregnancy or in the newborn period, and is not due to oxygen deprivation of the baby during labor. Cerebral palsy is defined by the National Institutes of Health as a non-progressive motor disorder of early infant onset involving one or more limbs, with resulting muscular spasticity or paralysis. It is rare, affecting 1-2/1000 births per year. The greatest pregnancy risk factor for cerebral palsy is preterm birth.

Intrapartum hypoxia is defined as a decrease in the baby's blood oxygen level, caused by a sustained low (i.e. sixty beats per minute) or severe and repetitive drops in the heart rate. Such abnormal heart rates must persist for ten to thirty minutes or more to affect the fetus. Intrapartum hypoxia cannot be *diagnosed* by an abnormal fetal heart rate. It can only be *suspected* by an abnormal fetal heart rate. Diagnosis of intrapartum hypoxia is made by sampling the baby's blood from a scalp sample during labor, or an umbilical cord sample immediately after delivery. Such blood sampling is not routinely done unless there is a question about fetal status during labor, or if the baby appears to be having difficulty shortly after birth.

Your ob provider will act on an abnormal fetal heart rate if it threatens to cause the baby intrapartum hypoxia long before any short term or long term harm is done. Your ob provider cares about you and your baby, and they care about their own career. They don't want you to have a bad outcome.

Because continuous monitoring during labor has not proven to be of clear benefit over intermittent auscultation, many labor units and ob providers have formally or informally adopted a protocol of intermittent fetal monitoring with the cardiotocodynamometer or a fetal Doppler. Monitoring may be conducted less frequently, i.e. every fifteen minutes to hour, in early labor when there is little stress to the baby; and more frequently, i.e. every five minutes, or after every contraction, or continuously, during the more strenuous later stages of labor and during pushing. Your ob provider will make decisions about frequency and type of fetal monitoring depending on the progress of your labor and your baby's response to the stress of labor.

> **A large body of evidence involving tens of thousands of births has shown that less than five percent of cerebral palsy results from events during labor, and the actual percentage may be close to zero.**

Internal Monitors

Fetal heart rate and contractions can be more accurately determined inside the uterus versus from external monitors placed on the abdomen. Usually internal monitors are used to better evaluate a problem with the fetal heart rate, or with the strength of the uterine contractions.

Fetal Scalp Electrode (FSE)

A fetal scalp electrode is a spiral shaped wire, about 3/8 inch in diameter and 1/8 inch "deep" that is rotated into the fetal scalp skin over a bony part of the fetal head. Scalp electrodes are not placed over the fontanelles (soft spots) of the head. This device penetrates *only the skin*, not the bone, brain, or other deep tissues. It senses fetal heart rate with more detail and accuracy than an external Doppler. A fetal scalp electrode may be used in situations where the fetal heart rate cannot be well detected; for example if the mother's abdomen is so thick the fetal heart can't be heard well through fatty tissue; or of there is concern about drops in the fetal heart rate and how they are timed with maternal contractions. Fetal scalp electrodes are safe and do not cause any damage to the baby's skull or brain.

Intra-Uterine Pressure Catheter (IUPC)

An internal uterine pressure catheter is a two-foot long tube or wire with a pressure sensing device integrated within the tip. It is placed using a stiff plastic guide positioned at the entrance of the dilated cervix. The catheter is introduced through the cervix next to the baby, and passed alongside the baby such that the tip is between the middle to top of the uterus. The plastic guide is pulled off by means of a slit along its side. The entire three foot length of the catheter does not reside in the uterus—only enough to achieve proper positioning. This device allows for much more accurate assessment of strength, frequency and duration of uterine contractions.

In comparison, external uterine pressure sensors can only measure frequency and duration of contractions, and are relatively imprecise. The strength of contractions measured by external pressure sensors can be affected by how tight the abdominal bands are cinched, the size of the mother's abdomen, and how much body fat she's carrying. Intra-uterine pressure catheters (IUPC's) are not affected by these variables.

What will labor be like?

Admission and Early Labor

Your ob provider will probably direct you to proceed to the birth unit if you are experiencing the following:

1) Regular contractions, occurring at least or less than every five minutes, and becoming progressively stronger and persisting for an hour or more.
2) Your water breaks.

3) You have continuous bright red vaginal bleeding.
4) You haven't felt the baby move.

Admission to the hospital

As you check in to the hospital you will be asked to register—provide your demographic and insurance information. Some hospitals and birth centers allow for preregistration to get this paperwork done during pregnancy, but before you actually present in labor.

Once registered, you will go to the labor unit. In the unit, a labor nurse will likely direct you to change into a hospital gown and place you on the fetal monitor for initial assessment of the baby's status and contractions. The labor nurse may check your cervix for dilation if you are experiencing regular contractions. She will then report on your assessment to your ob provider, most likely via phone. A labor nurse is trained to make a diagnosis of labor. Your midwife or doctor does not need to be present to determine whether or not you are in labor. There are many "false starts" and if your ob provider had to come in to see each pregnant patient every time they came into the hospital, he or she would never leave the hospital.

If you are diagnosed as being in labor (having regular uterine contractions accompanied by softening, thinning, and dilation of the cervix) you will likely be admitted. If you are diagnosed with false labor or prodromal labor, you may be discharged and instructed when to return.

Wearing your own clothes

Labor staff and hospitals usually have no problem with you wearing your own clothes, such as a gown, robe, bra, and socks during labor. However, labor makes a mess. Your attire will get soaked with amniotic fluid, blood, possibly vomit, urine and feces. So it's a good idea to take advantage of any gown, robe, and "booties" the labor unit provides. Whether or not to wear a bra is up to you. Once the baby is born, the bra will come off so the baby can try to latch on to the nipple and commence breast-feeding.

Walking and Eating

During early labor, after the initial assessment of you and the baby's status, you will probably be encouraged to walk around the labor unit or hospital. Walking may or may not facilitate labor, but it does at least provide something to do while waiting for labor to intensify. Many hospitals and ob providers will allow you to eat in early labor because it could be several hours or a day before you actually deliver.

Most women vomit at some point in labor, when the contractions intensify and the cervix dilates more rapidly. So whatever you eat in early labor, keep in mind you may be seeing it again in a different and less appetizing form later on.

If your water is broken you will continue to leak fluid—water, mucus and blood—throughout labor. The labor nurse will give you a very sexy "diaper" to contain the fluid as you walk about the unit.

Early Labor Contractions

As labor builds, the upper muscular part of the uterus contracts so as to cause the lower part of the uterus and cervix to soften, thin and dilate. With early labor contractions, your upper abdomen may or may not become hard and painful. Simultaneously, you may experience pressure or cramping in your lower abdomen and pelvis. Early labor contractions feel somewhat like menstrual cramps. Most babies begin labor with the head facing to one side or another, but if your baby is facing straight out (occiput posterior), with the roundest part of the head against your spine, you will experience more pressure and pain in your back ("back labor").

Walking and use of a hot tub or shower is a great way to manage discomfort of early labor.

Active Labor Contractions

Once your cervix is fully thinned out, the rate of dilation of the cervix accelerates. Your contractions may go from being five minutes apart to being one to two minutes apart. You may not be able to catch your breath between contractions during this phase of labor as they progress from mild to moderate to strong. At their peak intensity you won't be able to indent your uterus or abdomen by pressing with your finger during a strong contraction. Strong contractions are also accompanied by intense pain in the pelvis and/or lower back. As the baby moves down the birth canal you'll also experience pressure on the pubic bone, vagina, and rectum.

Walking, Swiveling, Rocking, "Doing the Ball"

There are several non-medical options to manage pain in this phase of labor. Pain medications will be addressed later in this chapter. You can still make use of walking, or bracing yourself against the edge of a bed or wall and swiveling your hips in a circle. Remaining upright gives you the advantage of allowing gravity to work with you rather than against you. It may also facilitate the proper flexion, descent, and internal rotation of the baby's head so your labor proceeds as normally as possible (see "Science Notes").

You may want to sit on a labor ball (a large rubber ball like an exercise ball) to support you while you rock and swivel your hips. A rocking chair can also serve this purpose but is less versatile.

A hot shower or hot tub may still be your friend at this stage, especially if you have back labor.

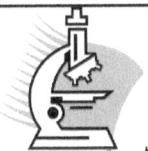

Science Notes: Rotation and Descent of the Baby in Labor:

The "Tuck" and "Roll"

Most babies begin labor facing one side or the other, with the spine along the mother's left or right side. During labor the baby undergoes three important maneuvers in the birth canal which determine whether you will have a normal or long labor, or in some cases will need assistance with delivery by vacuum, forceps or C-section. These maneuvers are **flexion**, **internal rotation** and **extension**.

Flexion (the "tuck") occurs at the beginning of labor and as the head enters the pelvis. As the baby descends, it is very important the neck flex so that the chin touches the chest. This allows the smallest diameter of the head to enter and traverse the pelvis. Hyper-extension of the neck can stop the progress of labor. Extreme extensions of the head can result in abnormal presentations such as a brow (forehead presenting) or face (full face presenting). Often these fetal presentations cannot deliver vaginally.

It is also important for the chin of the baby to be centered over the sternum, and not angled toward one shoulder or another. If angled, it produces **asynclitism** in which the head does not enter the pelvis "square" but rather with the head tilted too far to one shoulder, increasing the diameter that must fit through the birth canal. This slows labor.

Internal Rotation (the "roll") occurs after the baby's head has entered the pelvis. It is a rotation of the head from facing sideways to facing your spine. This position is called "occiput anterior" meaning the occiput (back of the head) is anterior (toward your front). Sometimes the baby rotates such that it faces your pubic bone instead of spine. If this occurs it is called "occiput posterior". Also known as "sunny side up", this position slows labor as the neck remains too extended and a larger diameter of the head must fit through the pelvis. Babies in the occiput posterior position often need assistance delivering with vacuum, forceps or C-section.

When the baby is deep in the birth canal, after most of internal rotation has taken place, *extension* is the next maneuver which allows the baby's head to move past your pubic bone. As the neck naturally extends the roundest part of the back of the head slides under the pubic bone and reaches the internal surface of the labia. Further extension and expulsion of the baby lead to "crowning" of the head.

Crowning occurs when enough of the head protrudes through the labia to produce a round stretching of the labia, about the diameter of a baseball.

In the *occiput anterior* position, when the baby's facing your back, once crowning occurs, the rest of the head follows easily within about a minute or less. After the head comes out, it is facing the floor with the chin pointing towards one of the baby's shoulders. Inside the birth canal, the baby's shoulders are still "sideways", aligned with your front to back axis (pubic bone to tail bone). The head naturally turns to one side or another such that it assumes a neutral position relative to the baby's breastbone. This is called *external rotation* and *restitution*.

In the *occiput posterior* position, the neck is already extended, so it doesn't slide under the pubic bone as easily as if the baby is in the occiput anterior position. This can cause the baby to get stuck in the birth canal, necessitating assistance with forceps, vacuum, or C-section. Babies delivered from the occiput posterior position often have a lot of facial bruising due to the face sliding against the maternal pubic bone, instead of the soft muscular back part of the vagina.

Notes on Photographs: In all the following pictures, the "baby" is a doll used for prenatal classes. The pelvis is a plastic model of a pelvis. The "perineum" is a cloth cover that fits over the model pelvis to simulate the soft tissues of the vagina and perineum. The "pregnant" woman is the author wearing a special suit. The birth attendants are a certified nurse midwife and a labor nurse. All photographs were taken by Doug Ellis, professional photographer.

Positions of the Baby in the Uterus

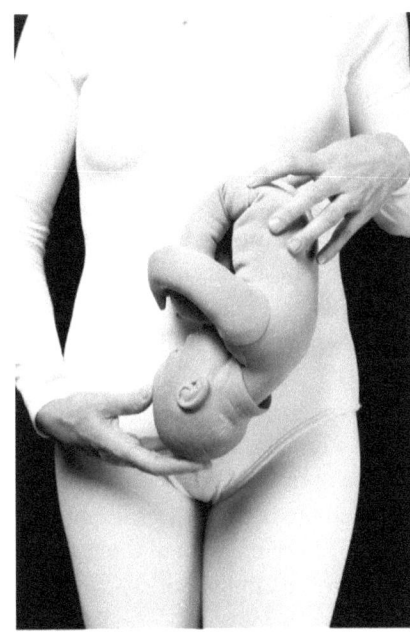

Left: Most babies enter labor facing to the side. Ideally, the head flexes so the chin is "tucked" onto the chest. With the chin tucked to chest, the smallest head circumference possible enters the pelvis. In the "**occiput anterior**" position the back of the head faces out towards mom's front.

Right: As the baby descends into the pelvis it **rotates** to face more toward mom's back. In the process of rotating the head flexes closer to the chest and makes it easier for the baby to enter the bony pelvis.

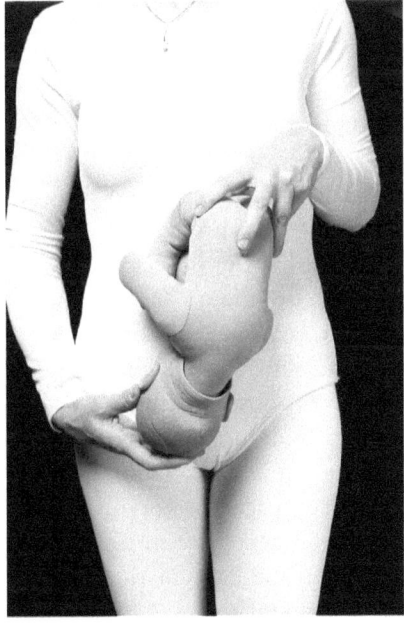

Positions of the Baby in the Uterus, continued ...

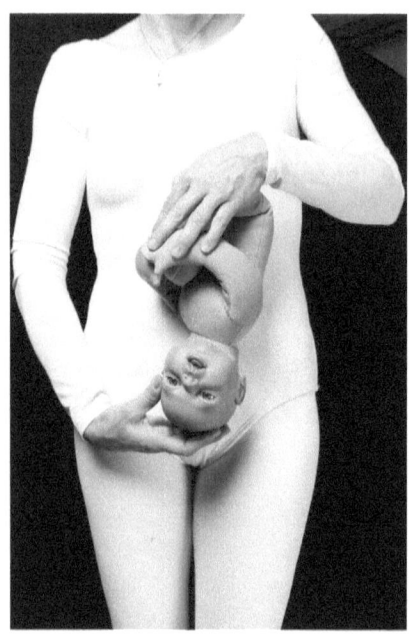

Left: This is the **occiput posterior** ("sunny side up") position. In this position the baby's head cannot flex as much. By remaining more extended, a larger circumference of the head enters the pelvis during labor. The back of the head "occiput" can press against the maternal spine and sacrum. This results in greater back pain compared to the occiput anterior position. Babies who remain in the occiput posterior position throughout pushing often are born with bruised faces due to the pressure of the face on the mom's pubic bone.

Right: In the occiput posterior position the head can actually become more **extended** throughout labor. The back of the head "catches" on mom's lower spine and sacral promontory (see pelvis illustration). This can prevent further descent of the baby into the pelvis, resulting in either **labor arrest** (stoppage) of cervical dilation and descent; or delivery of the baby in the "**face presentation**".

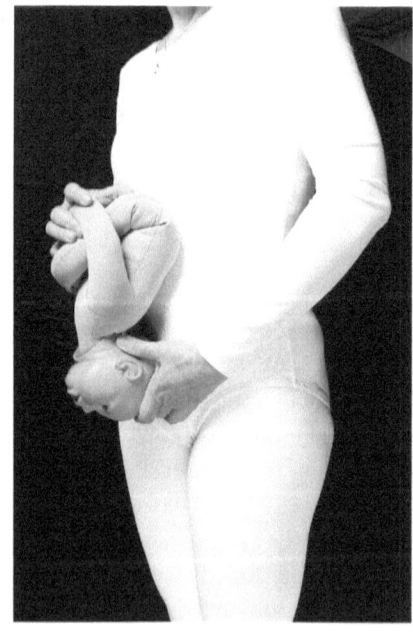

Positions of the Baby in the Uterus, continued ...

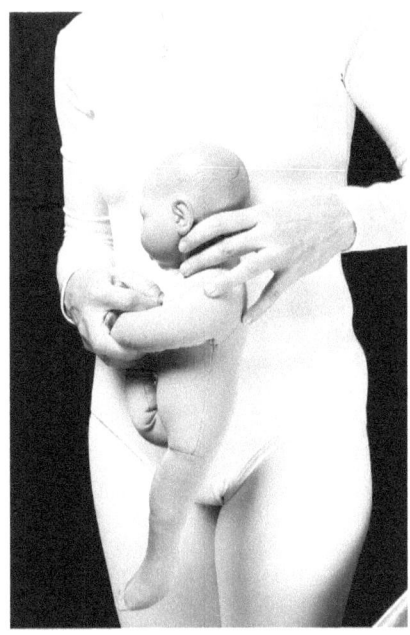

Left: This is the **footling breech** position. One foot is down and extended while the other is tucked. In a **double footling breech** position, both feet are down. In a **frank breech** position the fetal buttocks are the lowest part and the fetal hips are flexed so both feet are near the head. In a **complete breech** position, the baby sits in the uterus with the legs flexed and crossed at the ankles. The buttocks and feet are the lowest parts of the baby.

Right: This is an extreme version of the occiput posterior position, the face position. Babies can only deliver vaginally in the face position if the chin is toward the front of mom. Face presentations occur in about 1/1000 births; whereas the occiput posterior position occurs in about twenty percent of births.

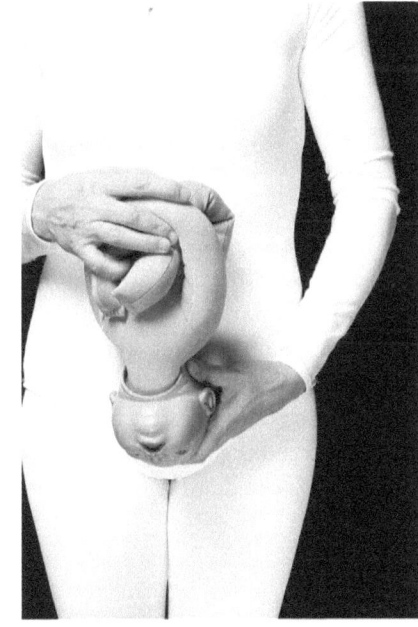

Important Diameters of the Fetal Head

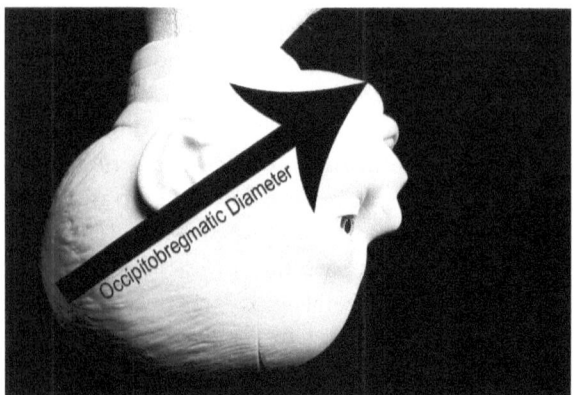

Left: The **occipito-bregmatic diameter** is the distance from the back of the head to the chin. It is the longest diameter of the fetal head and the one that causes the most trouble in the **occiput posterior** position.

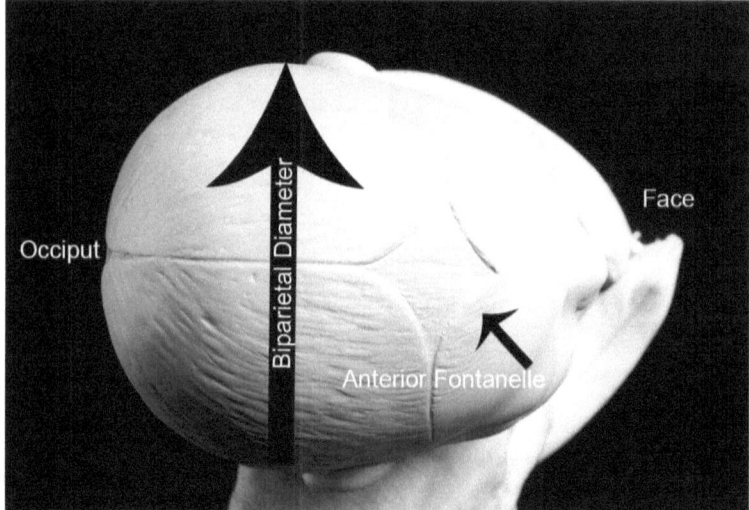

Above: The **biparietal diameter** is the widest point across the head. It is usually about nine to ten centimeters in the term infant. The diamond-shaped **anterior fontanelle** is the front "soft spot". The **occiput** is the rounded back of the head. The **posterior fontanelle** is not well seen in this picture, but looks similar to the anterior fontanelle, except it is triangular-shaped and located at the back of the head ("occiput").

Pelvic Anatomy

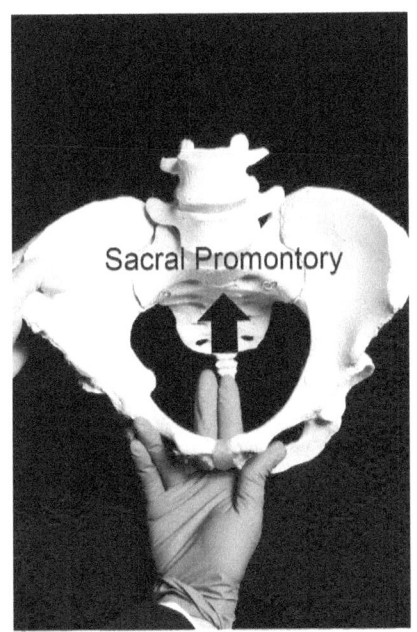

Left: The pelvis as viewed "from above". The **sacral promontory** is the rounding of the lower spine as it curves into the pelvis. The **hip bones** are the "wing-like" areas on the sides and the **pubic symphysis** is an area of cartilage at the front of the pelvis (bottom of picture). The pubic symphysis connects the two halves of the pelvis in front and allows for stretching in pregnancy labor.

The birth attendant's hand is shown as it would be if she were assessing the pelvis for "adequacy" or examining the cervix. Her fingers do not reach the sacral promontory, thus the pelvis is very "roomy" from front to back.

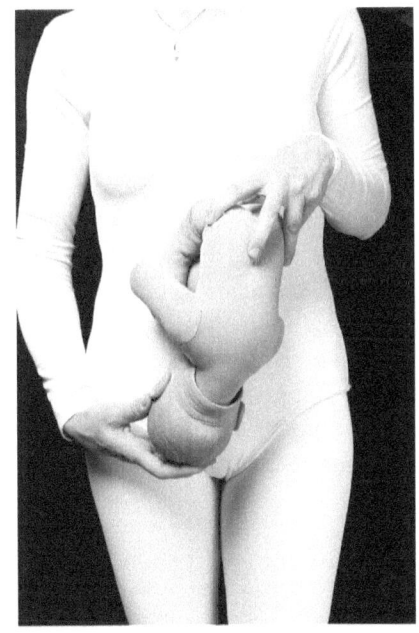

Right: The pelvis of the woman standing here is oriented similar to the picture above. The **pubic symphysis** actually angles downward in the standing position.

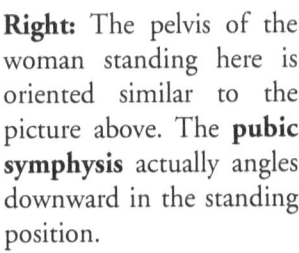

Pelvic Anatomy, continued …

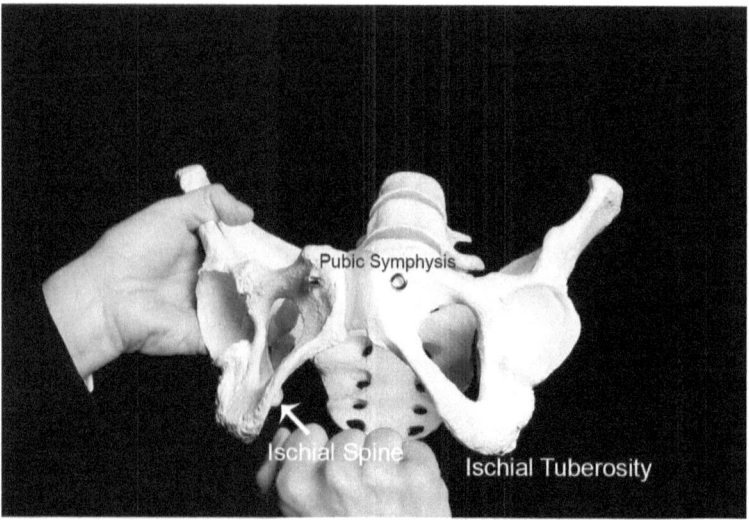

Above: : The pelvis as oriented in the reclining position. The **pubic symphysis** is shown at the top (grey area is supposed to represent cartilage).

The **ischial spines** (only one seen) are indicated by the white arrow. The distance between the ischial spines is the narrowest point the baby must navigate. It is also the reference for determining **station** or how far down in the pelvis the head is located. If the **biparietal diameter** of the head is at the level of the ischial spines, this is considered "zero station". Station is described as "plus" if it's beyond the ischial spines, and "minus" if the biparietal diameter has not reached the ischial spines.

The birth attendant is holding her fist between the two **ischial tuberosities**. These are the "butt bones" or the bony prominences upon which you rest when you sit upright. The distance between the ischial tuberosities roughly approximates the distance between the ischial spines. If this distance is greater than ten centimeters, the pelvis is considered "adequate" from side-to-side for vaginal delivery.

Fetal Monitors and Intra-Uterine Pressure Monitors

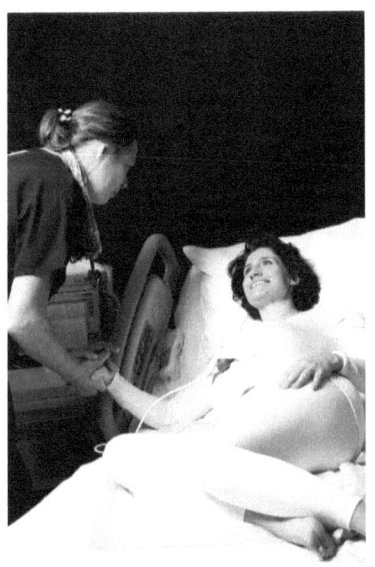

Left: The nurse (dressed in dark) has placed **external monitors** on the mother's abdomen. The one at the top of the abdomen is the "toco" and monitors contractions. The one at the bottom (hidden by the woman's hip) is the "**EFM**" or **external fetal monitor**.

The nurse is congratulating this woman for finding the labor ward, but you can tell from this mother's facial expression, she is not in labor. She is smiling and relaxed …

Right: An **intrauterine pressure catheter (IUPC)** is introduced into the pelvis with a "straw-like" applicator that is slit down the side. After the IUPC is positioned to the satisfaction of the birth attendant, the applicator is removed by pulling it off the catheter.

In the uterus the IUPC rests alongside and around the baby. It does not harm the baby. IUPC's directly measure the pressure in the uterus with a pressure sensor. IUPC's are used to assess strength, frequency, and duration of contractions when labor seems slowed or stopped.

An IUPC can help the birth attendant decide if oxytocin is necessary and can help her choose the dose of oxytocin.

Adequacy of contractions must be established before the decision is made to proceed to cesarean delivery.

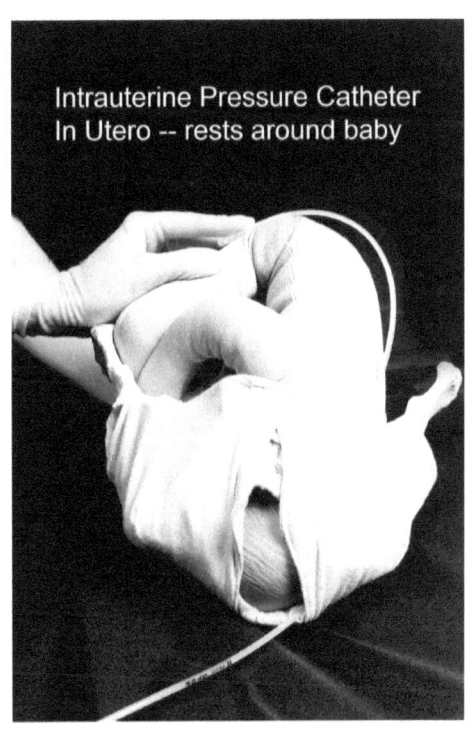

Intrauterine Pressure Catheter
In Utero -- rests around baby

Fetal Monitors, continued ...

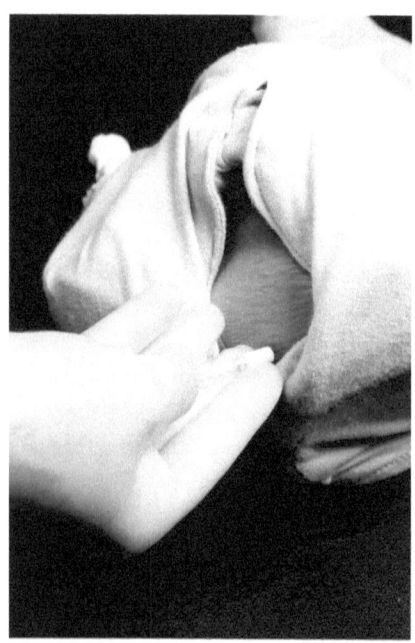

Left: The birth attendant introduces a **fetal scalp electrode (FSE)** to improve detection of the fetal heart rate. The FSE is applied to the fetal head with an applicator, similar to that of an IUPC applicator. The FSE is rotated once to anchor it in the fetal scalp skin, and the applicator is removed.

FSE's do not hurt the baby. The birth attendant is careful not to insert an FSE on a fontanelle, but even if she did, it can't penetrate the skin deep enough to harm the brain.

Right: This is a close-up view of an FSE. The metal wire does not penetrate the skin very deeply. It is rotated into the arm skin of this demonstrator. It does not hurt, and is actually barely perceptible.

The wire transmits the fetal heart rate signal and the clear sheath on the outside is the applicator, which will be removed once the FSE wire is anchored to the fetal scalp.

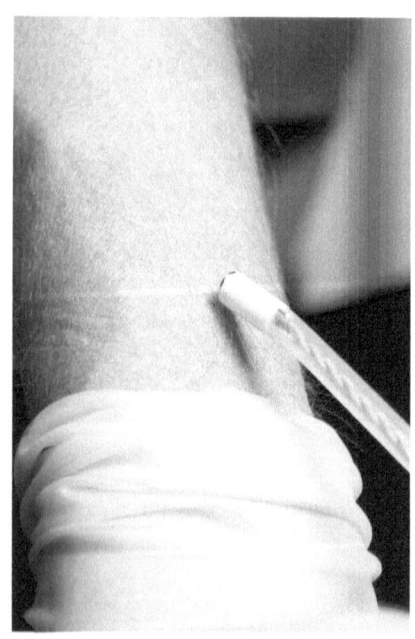

The Faces of Labor

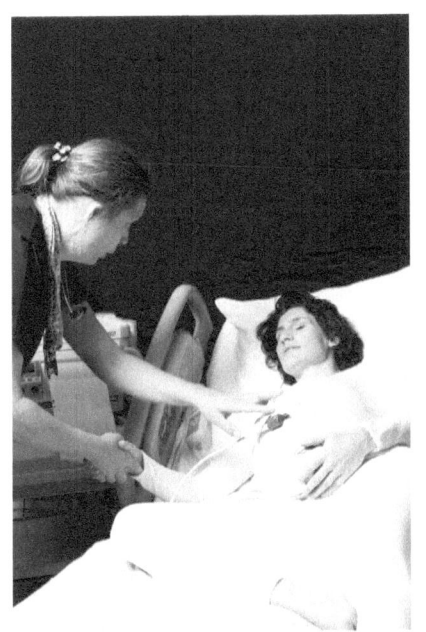

Left: Active Labor.

Whereas the woman pictured above was smiling and relaxed, this woman's expression is one of concentration. She is using breathing exercises to manage the pain.

The nurse or birth attendant supports her by holding her hand and offering words of encouragement.

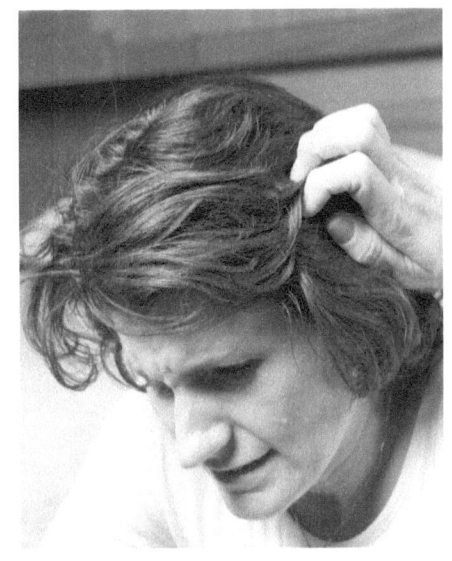

Right: Transition.

This woman is "**in transition**". She is undergoing rapid cervical dilation in the later phase of active labor.

Her expression tells us she is in more pain and experiencing pelvic pressure.

Positions for Active Labor

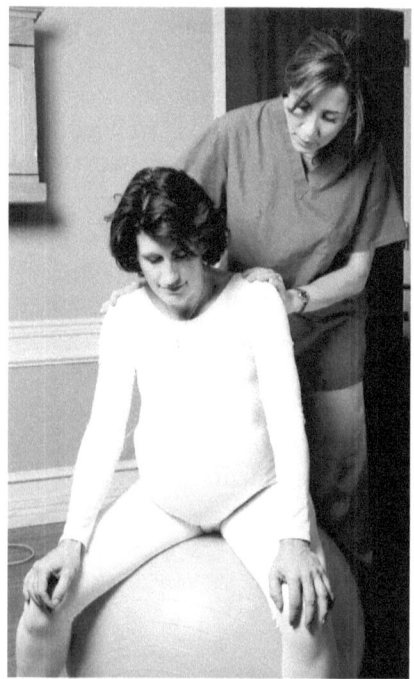

Besides walking, standing upright, or reclining, there are many other positions helpful for management of the active phases of labor.

Left: "On the Ball": Laboring on an inflatable rubber ball assists with pain management, especially in active labor and transition. It can also relieve some of the pain of back labor.

Below: The **"hip swivel"** or pelvic rock helps with active labor, transition, and with managing labors in which the baby is in the occiput posterior position—it eases rotation of the baby.

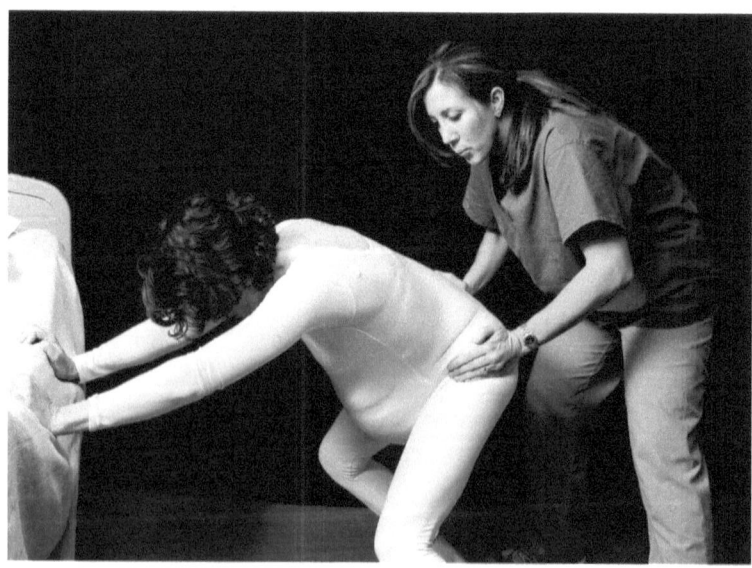

Positions for Active Labor continued ...

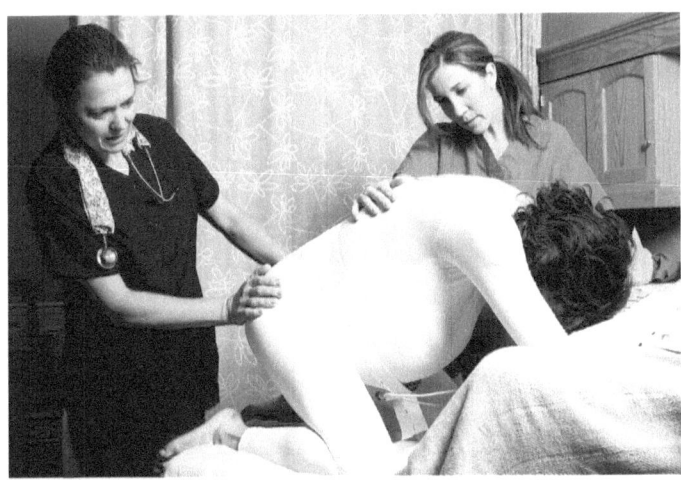

Above: "Hands and Knees" position is useful for many situations. It relieves pain of back labor. It can help rotate a baby from the occiput posterior position to the occiput anterior position. It can alleviate a low fetal heart rate by reducing pressure on the fetal umbilical cord.

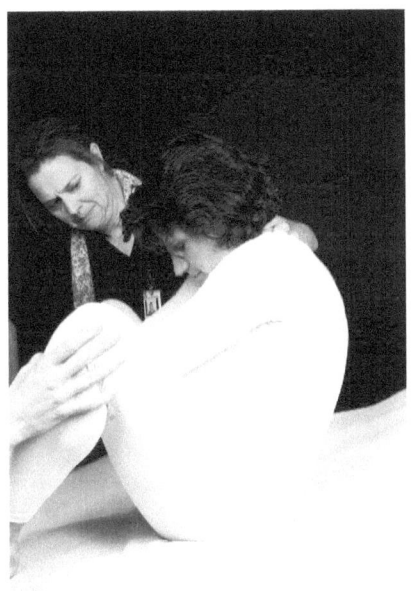

Left: The **C Position** is an essential position for labor and pushing. The mother curves her spine around the baby. Her chin touches her chest; her knees are up toward her chest. This rotates the pubic bone upward and opens the pelvis. It actually increases the distance between the sacral promontory and the pubic bone by as much as two centimeters (about one inch). The C position can be done sitting, squatting, or reclining.

Positions for Pushing

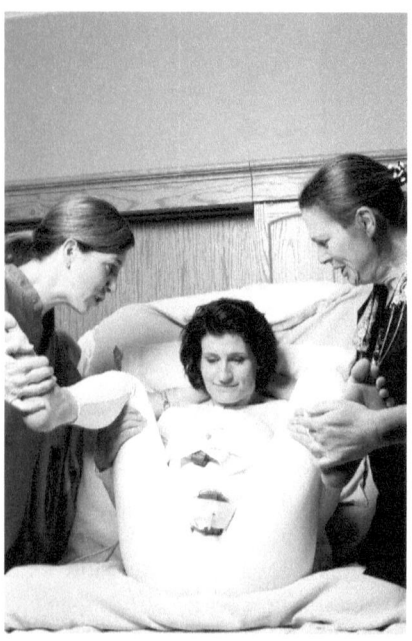

Left: Pushing in the **C Position, semi-upright** with pillows to support the back. The birth attendants are supporting the legs, but the mother does all the "heavy lifting" by grasping the backs of her legs and pulling her knees up, out, and toward her chest.

This position opens the pelvis front-to-back and side-to-side. It can add an inch of room front-to-back and can make all the difference in getting a baby out whose occiput posterior or has big shoulders.

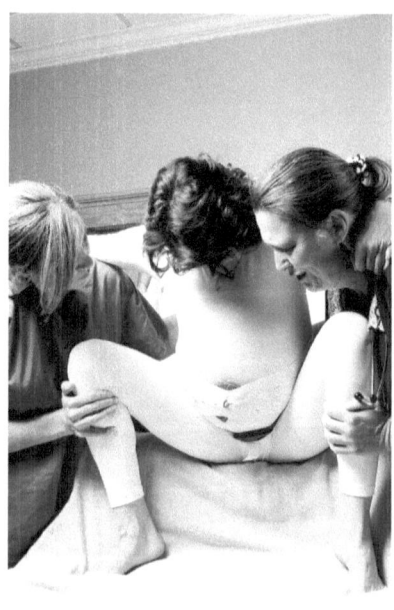

Right: Pushing in the squatting position. Mother is resting on birth attendants. However, birth attendants should not bear mother's weight for more than a few minutes because it can lead to back injury.

Positions for Pushing, continued …

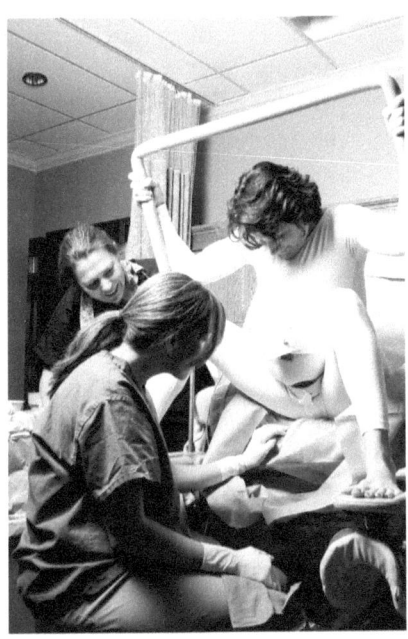

Left: Pushing in the squatting position with a **squat bar**. If this is available it is much safer than leaning on birth attendants.

The vertical orientation of the squatting position makes use of gravity in getting the baby delivered.

Below: Pushing with a towel, "Tug of War". This position with the mother and a birth assistant each pulling the ends of a twisted towel, helps ease delivery of a baby in the occiput posterior position. Sometimes it actually rotates the baby to the occiput anterior position.

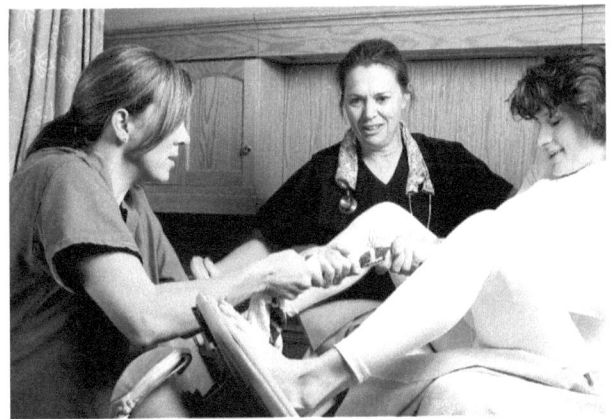

Supporting the Perineum

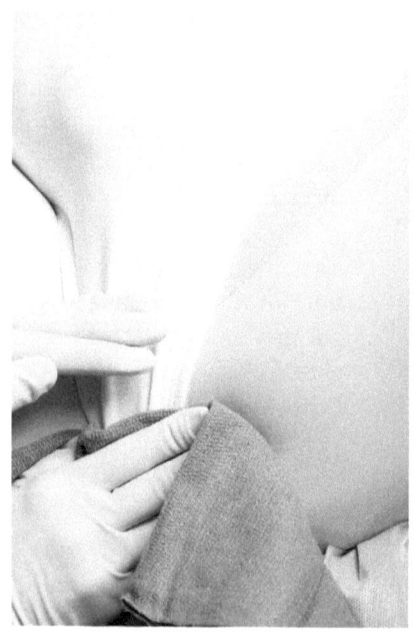

Left: The birth attendant is showing how to support the perineum. The baby is not in the picture. She supports the perineum by exerting gentle pressure on the skin on either side of the vaginal opening and squeezing her fingers and thumb toward each other to create stretch on the outer tissue and alleviate stretch near the vaginal opening. This can reduce the chances of a vaginal tear.

Right: Most women tear with delivery of the posterior shoulder as it comes through the vagina. It is essential to provide perineal support as the posterior shoulder is delivering to minimize the chance of tearing.

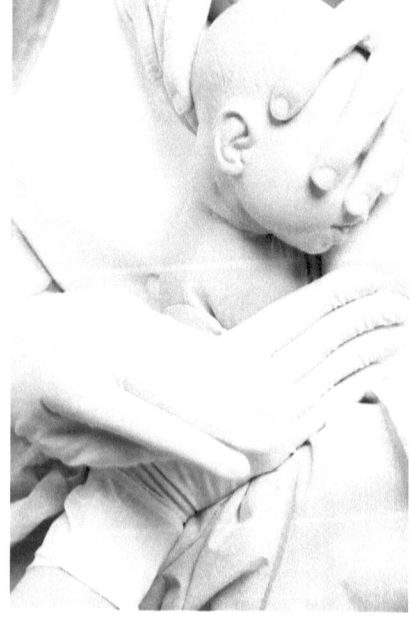

In this photo the model mother is delivering a model baby and the birth attendant is providing perineal support as the back shoulder passes the perineum.

Delivery Maneuvers

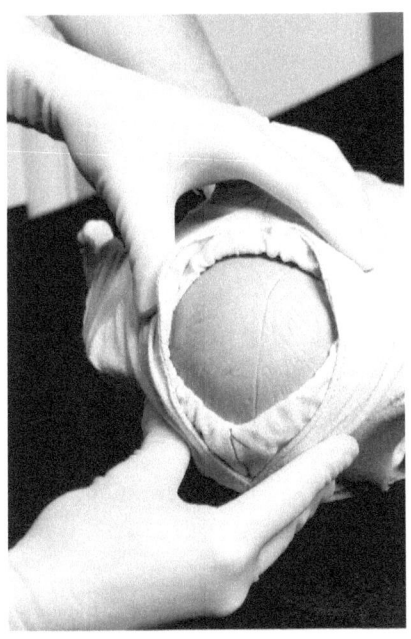

Left: Crowning. This is a pelvic model demonstrating crowning. Crowning occurs when the head fully distends the perineum and opens the labia. It means the baby's almost here!

The birth attendant is supporting the perineum as the head crowns.

Right: Hand position for delivering the head. This shows the birth attendant gently grasping the sides of the head with **flat opened hands.** She can then exert **downward pressure** to ease the **anterior shoulder** out; followed by **upward pressure** to ease the **posterior shoulder** out.

Once the head is delivered the mouth and nose can be suctioned , if necessary, with a bulb suction device to remove mucus and fluid.

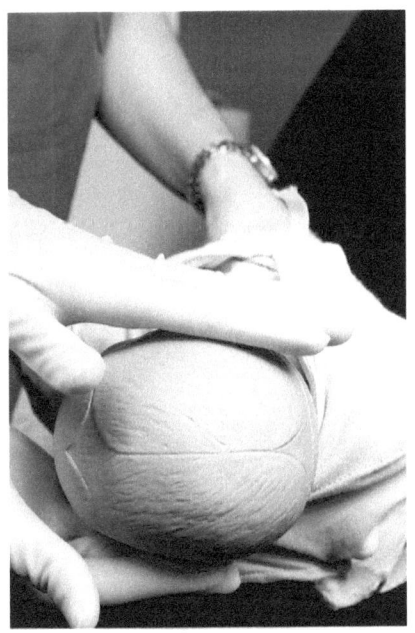

Delivery Maneuvers, continued ...

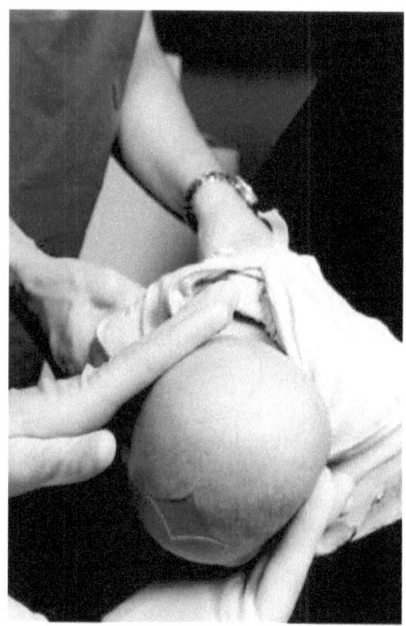

Left: Often the head delivers facing downward (occiput anterior). It then rotates to one side or the other. The birth attendant can support the head as it rotates.

Right: The head is rotating to face the maternal right side. The birth attendant supports the head with a hand on either side.

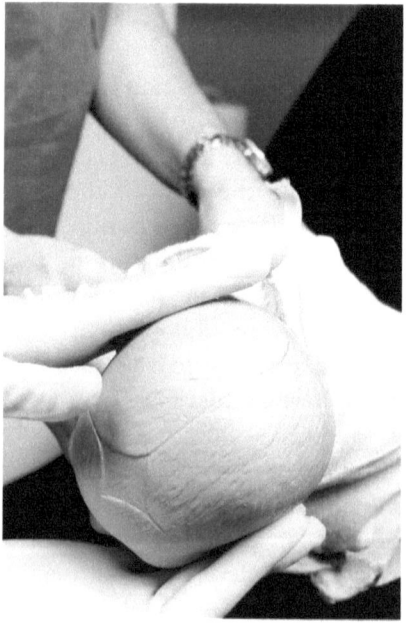

Delivery Maneuvers, continued ...

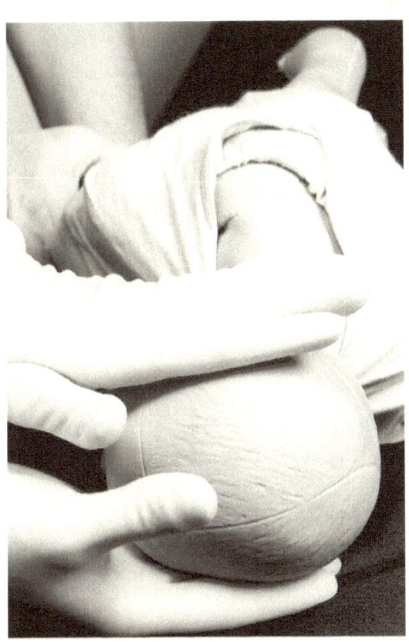

Left: The **anterior shoulder** is delivered by exerting **gentle downward traction** on the head. The shoulder slides under the pubic bone.

Right: The **posterior shoulder** is delivered by supporting the baby's head and neck with one hand, while the other hand supports the perineum as the shoulder passes through the vaginal opening.

The birth attendant exerts **gentle upward traction** to deliver the back shoulder.

The birth attendant is supporting the head with fingers on each side of the head; she's not grasping the baby by the neck.

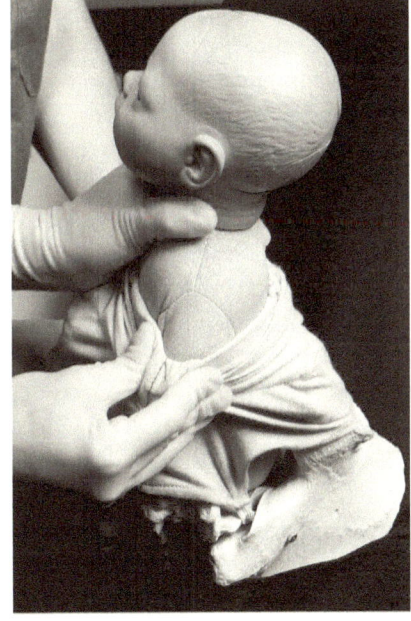

Back Labor

Back labor is felt in the lower back. It usually arises when the baby is in the occiput posterior position, "sunny side up", with the baby facing toward your pubic bone instead of toward your

> **Twenty percent of babies enter labor in the occiput posterior position.**

lower spine and sacrum. About twenty percent of babies proceed through labor in the occiput posterior position. Babies in the "sunny side up" position cause back labor because the most protuberant part of the head, the occiput or back of the head, is pressed against your lower spine and sacrum. In this position the baby's head cannot flex and "tuck" so it will exert more pressure on both your back and your pubic bone as the baby descends the birth canal.

The occiput posterior position results in a larger diameter of the head moving through the birth canal. When the baby faces your back, the occiput anterior position, the diameter of the head moving through the birth canal is ear-to-ear, roughly ten centimeters. However, when the baby is in the occiput posterior position, the diameter of the head that must traverse the birth canal is the chin-to-crown. This diameter can be as much as two centimeters, almost an inch, greater than the ear-to-ear diameter: a bigger object must fit through the same bone structure of your pelvis. Labor with the baby in the occiput posterior position usually takes longer, often needs assistance in delivery with forceps, vacuum, or C-section and can result in more damage to your pelvic floor, i.e. a bigger tear in the vagina and perineum.

The occiput posterior position will usually be diagnosed by your ob provider or labor nurse with a cervical exam. Your abdomen may also have a "double hump" which is the baby's folded arms and legs facing out, rather than the smooth back or side.

The occiput posterior position can also produce a characteristic pattern of uterine contractions known as "coupling". This pattern consists of brief weak contractions in pairs, rather than one sustained forcible uterine contraction. It is a less effective means of moving the baby through the pelvis, but it's not completely ineffectual and it doesn't mean you're consigned to a long labor or a C-section. If the baby rotates out of the occiput posterior position, coupling can evolve into a normal labor pattern.

Back labor is particularly uncomfortable, because in addition to pain from contractions, it can feel like the baby is "grinding" against your lower spine, sacrum, and rectum. Pelvic rocking and use of the labor ball can be especially helpful in managing the discomfort of back labor. Hands and knees position while rocking your hips can sometimes help the baby "roll" or make the internal rotation so it faces your side or back instead of pubic bone.

Deep massage with hands or even a rolling pin can provide distraction and relief from intense back labor. Allowing the shower to run on your back, or using a jetted tub can aid in management of back labor.

If the baby remains in the occiput position until you are completely dilated, there are some techniques to help the baby descend and may prevent you from needing assistance with vacuum, forceps or C-section. These will be discussed in the section on "Pushing".

Asynclitism or "Tilted Head"

Asynclitism can present the same hurdles as the occiput posterior position. Asynclitism results when the baby's ear is tilted more toward one shoulder, rather than being in a neutral position. One side of the neck is extended, and one side is flexed. It can produce back labor

> **Asynclitism is the "tilting" of the head so the ear is closer to the shoulder, rather than in a neutral position.**

because the temporal region or upper side of the head and shoulder grind along the sacrum, rather than the back of the head, as in the occiput posterior position. Asynclitism can prolong cervical dilation and descent of the baby. Sometimes it needs assistance in delivery with forceps or vacuum to "straighten out" the head. Often the mere application of the forceps, without actual traction on them will be enough to straighten out the head and result in successful vaginal delivery. Your ob provider may also be able to maneuver the head to a neutral position with her hand.

"Transition"

Transition is the out-of-control (OOC) phase: when you evolve from being the fantasy woman in the television labor, able to handle labor with aplomb—white dress, makeup, pedi-

> **Transition is the "Point of No Return".**

cure, and hair-do intact, to being the girl whose head spins as she hurls curse words and spews pea-soup vomit at everyone in range. Transition feels like the point of no return, you're never quite ready for it, no matter how much breathing you've practiced, childbirth classes you've attended, and reading you've done. This is when you may change your mind about "natural childbirth" with "no pain medications".

If you're in your labor room and you hear women screaming from the other labor rooms, they're in transition or pushing. Don't worry—that will soon be you. During transition your cervix quickly dilates and the fetal head descends rapidly. Transition can start at any dilation, especially if this is not your first labor. However, in first labors it usually hits when your cervix is six to seven centimeters dilated. You'll feel intense pressure on your back, pelvic muscles, vagina, pubic bone, and rectum. It basically feels like a freight train is trying to drive between your legs.

Transition isn't discussed in textbooks but most good labor nurses and ob providers recognize it by sight, sound and smell. When you hit transition *the baby is coming*.

The major goal of transition is: survive. This is when your "focal point" may come in handy. You may or may not have thought about pain medication before transition. If not, now is the time. Don't be afraid to ask for pain medicine or an epidural because these can really help ("save your life").

Every woman is a heroine and everyone gets a baby at the end and you don't get a blue ribbon or trumpet serenade for doing it without pain medication. If you walk the postpartum ward after everyone's delivered you won't see halos over the heads of the moms who did it without pain meds.

Pain Medication: Options

If you need pain meds it doesn't mean you're a "wimp". So many variables can affect how people experience pain. Every woman has different amounts of nerve fibers providing sensation to the uterus, cervix, and vagina. Women who do not need pain medications in labor may have fewer nerve fibers, or they may have pelvic shapes conducive to labor, or the baby may be small and in an easy position for delivery. Your labor will not be like your friend's or even your mother's or sister's labor. You don't have anything to prove. Do what you need to do.

Pain medications come in three forms: intravenous narcotics, epidural or spinal, and local skin or nerve blocks. Narcotics can be administered at any point in labor, and are sometimes used to differentiate false labor or prodromal labor from pre-labor. Epidural and spinal blocks are usually used for "active" labor and "pushing". Nerve blocks and local anesthesia are used for pushing or for repairs.

Intravenous Narcotics

Intravenous narcotics include drugs such as Fentanyl, Demerol, and Stadol. They are opiates and interact with the endorphin or pain relief receptors in your brain and nerve endings. Opiates

> **Narcan reverses the effects of opiates on the baby within seconds.**

can make you feel "high" or mildly sedated and may even let you sleep between contractions. Opiates are short-lived; most last one to two hours and have to be repeated at these intervals. However, one or two doses of intravenous opiates may be enough to get you through active labor or transition.

Opiates cross the placenta and affect the baby. If they are administered close to delivery, the baby may be "sleepy" and display sluggish respiratory effort. However, opiates are not harmful to the baby and any opiate effects in the newborn can be reversed by administering a drug called "Narcan". Narcan reverses the effects of opiates in the newborn, causing a baby having trouble breathing to exhibit improved respiratory effort.

Opiates can blunt the pain of contractions. Some women find opiates adequate for transition, others don't. If you need pain medication, have tried intravenous narcotics and found them ineffective, consider a regional anesthetic (epidural or spinal).

Regional Anesthetics: Epidural and Spinal

Epidurals

An epidural is pain medication administered via a thin tube called a catheter, similar to an intravenous catheter, only it goes into your back instead of a vein. It is usually placed by an anesthesiologist or nurse-anesthetist. Most ob providers are not trained to place epidurals.

The epidural catheter is introduced into the epidural space around the thick membrane covering the actual spinal cord. A bag like an I.V. is filled with numbing medicine such as "bupivicaine" (similar to what you might receive at the dentist) and/or a narcotic such as Fentanyl.

Epidurals have several advantages. Similar to I.V.'s they can allow for the continuous infusion of pain medication throughout labor. If you're stuck with a long labor or an induced labor, epidurals can provide uninterrupted pain relief for hours at a time. Epidurals can allow you to sleep through labor. If you're very tense, an epidural can allow you to relax and in some instances may facilitate descent of the baby through the pelvis.

Much less pain medication gets to the baby when you have an epidural or spinal versus intravenous pain medication. Scant medication makes it into your bloodstream to cross the placenta and affect the baby.

Research on epidurals and their effect on labor is controversial. The best studies show that epidurals do not increase the Cesarean section rate. They may prolong second stage, or pushing, but allowances are made for this by your ob provider in determining whether you may need assistance with delivery via forceps or C-section. Usually you're allowed an extra hour for pushing if you have an epidural, before deeming the second stage of your labor is abnormally long and in need of intervention. This approach varies somewhat from provider to provider, and may be affected by other factors complicating your labor such as an occiput posterior position or a large baby.

Complications from epidurals are rare. The most common side effect is a spinal headache and may affect $1/1,000$ to $1/10,000$ people who receive epidurals. This rate may vary depending on your provider. The anesthetist will probably also quote you complications such as nerve damage and paralysis, but these are extremely rare, less than $1/100,000$. I have never seen or heard of anyone with any long lasting complication of an epidural or spinal. A spinal headache results from too much spinal fluid "leaking" out of the epidural or spinal site. It can be treated by lying flat, administering intravenous fluid, or a "blood patch", which consists of drawing a tube of your own blood and injecting it into the space around the spine to replace a spinal fluid leak. Spinal headaches are infrequent and easily alleviated.

Sometimes an epidural can cause your blood pressure to drop during or shortly after it's initiated. This effect is reversed by administering intravenous fluid and ephedrine (a medication), which increases your blood pressure to normal. You might see the baby's heart rate drop for a few minutes if your blood pressure drops. Again this is mitigated by changing your position, giving you oxygen, intravenous fluids, and ephedrine. Decreases in the fetal heart rate related to epidurals are usually short-lived and of no long-term consequence to fetal well-being.

After you deliver, the epidural catheter is removed and it takes a few hours for the medicine to wear off.

You may have heard of a "walking epidural" in your prenatal classes, from friends, or reading. "Walking" epidurals are intended to provide pain relief, but still allow you the ability to move. This type of epidural is composed of mostly narcotic pain medication in the epidural solution, and very little numbing medicine. However, a walking epidural is a bit of a misnomer. Although you can move around with this type of epidural, it can blunt your balance receptors and make it difficult to actually "walk". Moreover, epidurals usually require numbing medicine such as bupivicaine or lidocaine to provide adequate relief of pain.

Spinals

A spinal is similar to an epidural, except it's a "one shot deal". A spinal is injected into the fluid around the spinal nerves, rather than along the sac that surrounds the spinal cord. Usually spinals are given late in labor and intended to last just for pushing. A spinal can be a better option than epidural if you are completely dilated and ready to push, but in need of pain relief to work with the labor.

Local Anesthesia and Nerve Blocks (Pudendals)

Local anesthesia is numbing medicine such as novacaine (lidocaine) or bupivicane injected into the skin of the vulva to provide anesthesia for crowning, for an episiotomy, or for repair of a tear or episiotomy. Local anesthetics are placed by your ob provider and last thirty to sixty minutes. They are great for short term relief of pain for a small area. Local anesthetics are not used to manage contraction pain or long labors.

Pudendal nerve blocks are local anesthetics (numbing medicines) injected into the nerves along each side of the pelvis that provides sensation to the labia, vulva and the lower vagina. A pudendal nerve block may be placed by your ob provider. Pudendal blocks last about an hour and can be used to alleviate pain with pushing, to provide pain relief for a vacuum or forceps delivery, or to provide pain relief for a repair.

Local anesthetics are short-lived, do not affect the baby, and have almost no complications.

Pushing (Second Stage of Labor)

Once your cervix is fully dilated, it's up to you. Oh—and the shape of your pelvis, position and size of the baby. But mostly, it's up to you.

You will know when your cervix is fully dilated and you are ready to push because you will feel intense pressure in the lower vagina and rectum, like you have the urge to have a bowel movement. This will be less so with an epidural, but you still may experience the sensation of pressure.

The basic maneuver of pushing is to bear down with your abdominal muscles, and relax your pelvic muscles as though you are going to have a bowel movement. Make use of your contractions, and push during the contractions, resting in-between. As your contraction builds, gather a big breath to fill your lungs with air. Then hold your breath, bear down for a count of ten seconds, take a quick breath in-between and push again. Try to push three times with each contraction.

Positioning during pushing is flexible—almost anything goes. You can push in semi-Fowler's position, seated with your head and shoulders elevated. You can also push in the squatting position; and many labor units have "squatting bars" that mount to the labor beds and give you a support to hang onto while pushing in this position. You can push in the hands and knees position. This may be helpful if you are trying to rotate the baby from the occiput posterior position so the baby faces your back. Pushing on one side can also help rotate a baby.

While anything goes during pushing, there are a couple of maneuvers that can help make birthing a baby easier. These are the "C-Position" and "Hips Flexed and Out". There's an elegant element of geometry involved in successful vaginal birth, especially when the baby is in the occiput posterior position, you have a large baby, or narrow pelvis.

The C Position

While squatting or lying on your back, tuck your chin to your chest, round your spine around your baby and rotate your pelvis forward. This is the C position. The C position orients the long axis of the baby toward your pelvis and directs the head toward the bony "inlet" of your pelvis. It opens the distance between your pubic bone and sacrum (lower spine) and it facilitates movement of the baby down the birth canal by enhancing internal rotation of the head and increasing the front-to-back area of the pelvis, thus allowing the baby more room.

Hips Flexed and Out

In the semi-supine or squatting position if you pull back your knees up and out it opens your pelvis, allowing easier passage of the baby. This maneuver pulls the pubic bone upward and away from your sacrum. Not only does this create more room in the pelvis from front-to-back, it also causes the pubic symphysis to slide up over the fetal head or shoulder. Sometimes this maneuver, and maintaining the C position while pushing can make the difference between delivering unassisted, or needing help with vacuum or forceps. The knees-back-and-out position also reduces the chance of shoulder dystocia, or trapping of the shoulder behind the pubic bone with possible injury to the baby's shoulder nerves.

Normal Duration of Second Stage

Normal second stage is defined as one hour. For your first baby if you don't have an epidural you may push anywhere from ten to sixty minutes. More than sixty minutes of pushing is considered "prolonged". With an epidural, you may push up to two hours before second stage is considered prolonged. Second or subsequent babies usually deliver faster in general, but this is not an absolute, as the fetal size and position and other factors impact the duration of labor.

Special Techniques for Delivering the Occiput Posterior or Asynclitic Baby

Twenty percent of you will have a baby in the occiput posterior position. Asynclitism affects about five percent. There are several techniques for you to manage or correct the occiput posterior and asynclitic baby. Fundamental are the C Position and Knees Flexed and Out. Don't forget these as they are your friends and may mean the difference between delivering unassisted versus assisted. However if these don't result in baby moving down the birth canal here are some other maneuvers you can try.

Pushing With a Towel: Tug of War

Although I feel empathy for my patient who's struggling with labor, it can give dad the opportunity to become more involved with labor with a little game of Tug of War to help mom deliver.

Use an assistant such as a family member with a strong back and arms. The father of the baby works great for this job, plus it gives him an appreciation for how much work labor can be. A labor nurse, doula or other assistant can suffice if she possesses the willingness, strength and energy for a major workout.

The object of this is to push in the C position with your feet braced against the stirrups while holding one end of a twisted towel or short thick rope. Your partner stands between your legs and provides counter traction. As you're pushing, pull back with as much force as you can on the towel, but do not arch your back. This accentuates the C position, rolls the pubic bone over the descending part of the baby, and multiplies your power. While you are pushing/pulling on the towel, your partner pulls on his end of the towel like you're in a game of Tug of War. His counter-traction again accentuates your C position and gives you added power. Your feet MUST be braced on something or this maneuver will be ineffective and you will merely slide down the bed or whatever surface on which you're pushing.

Hands and Knees

Laboring or pushing on your hands and knees will sometimes allow gravity to assist you in the internal rotation of the baby from an occiput posterior or side position to an occiput anterior position. It can be tough to maintain your C position but do your best to keep your chin to chest and spine curled around the baby.

Squatting

Squatting has the same effect on geometry of the pelvis and baby as the Tug of War position. However, you don't get the same force in this position as you do with the Tug of War. Squatting is most effective if you have use of a squatting bar which mounts to a labor bed and provides you support and leverage.

Do Not Despair

Sometimes despite all your efforts the shape of your pelvis or the size and position of the baby will conspire against you and you will need assistance with forceps, vacuum or C-section. *This is not a failure on your part.* It's simply the laws of physics.

The Baby Delivers (At Last)

Once the head is crowning you're home free. Crowning is when the baby's head is fully applied to your pelvic floor. You will recognize this because the vaginal opening will be dilated to greater than the diameter of a silver dollar and you will see this portion of the head protruding through the vulva and distending your perineum. The portion of the head you see is from above the forehead hair line to the crown of the head. During and subsequent to crowning your ob provider may place a hand on your perineum to give it some support and minimize tearing.

Further pushing efforts will completely propel the head through the vulva. During this time your ob provider may exert gentle pressure on the baby's head to flex it more and allow it to slide under your pubic bone with minimal chance of tearing the tissues at the front of the vulva near the urethral opening. Once the head is delivered your ob provider will have you push again to deliver the shoulders. The anterior shoulder, which is under your pubic bone, delivers first. Again, maintain your C position with Knees Up and Out because this rotates the pubic bone over the shoulder. Your ob provider may exert gentle downward traction with hands against the side of the baby's head to help you expel the anterior shoulder.

Delivery of the anterior shoulder is followed by delivery of the posterior shoulder, which is near your rectum and sacrum. Your ob provider may exert gentle upward traction on the head to facilitate delivery of the posterior shoulder.

Once the posterior shoulder has delivered the rest of the baby delivers and congratulations, you've done it! Welcome to parenthood!

Your ob provider may dry the baby a little, then place your baby on your tummy for you to meet and enjoy. Suspending the baby from the ankles and slapping the baby's bottom is a throwback to "ancient times" (the 1960's) and is no longer practiced.

Other birth attendants such as labor nurses may suction, dry, and stimulate the baby to get her to open her lungs, cry, and mobilize fluid and mucus from the airways. Touching the baby, rubbing her feet, drying her off, and suctioning her airway all prompt her to cry and take her first breaths.

Once you're holding your baby, your ob provider will clamp the cord and often ask the father or other relative to cut the cord. There is no hurry to clamp and cut the cord. Some ob providers wait until the cord has stopped pulsating to clamp it, others don't.

> **It is normal for your baby's hands and feet to be blue at birth and for several minutes afterward.**

It is normal for your baby's hands and feet to be blue at birth and for several minutes or longer afterward. Newborn circulation favors the vital organs, the brain, heart, and lungs, at the expense of the hands and feet. So your baby's blue hands and feet will gradually turn pink by five to ten minutes after birth, after the vital organs have been adequately oxygenated. The change will be slower if your baby is born at higher altitude.

If your baby needs extra help "getting started" he will be carried to the infant warmer to obtain whatever assistance he needs. This may include a little extra oxygen with a tube "blowing by the nose and mouth" or mask ventilation if the baby requires additional support. Sometimes babies who've undergone a stressful labor need this extra help to establish normal respiratory and cardiac function. Babies who need extra help at the beginning usually recover quickly and rarely exhibit any persistent effects of a stressful labor.

Tears vs. Episiotomy

Almost everyone will tear during birth and very few ob providers still do "routine episiotomies".

Most tearing occurs *after* crowning with delivery of the baby's lower face, neck, and posterior shoulder (the one facing your back). Tears are defined by the layers through which they extend. A **first degree** tear is just through the vaginal skin and perineum. A **second degree** tear is through the skin and underlying tissues such as the puborectalis and pubococcygeus muscles. A **third degree** tears extends partially or fully through the external anal sphincter; and a **fourth degree** tear extends into the rectum. These more extensive tears tend to occur with occiput posterior deliveries. Only five percent of women will have a third or fourth degree tear. All tears and episiotomies are repaired in layers, beginning with the deepest and proceeding to the most superficial. See "Science Notes" below for anatomy terms.

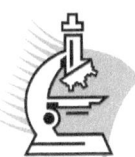

Science Notes: Anatomy of the Pelvic Floor

Your pelvic floor is your center of gravity. When standing upright, picture your pelvic floor as a bowl-shaped group of muscles contained within the bony pelvis. The "bottom" of the bowl is actually shaped like a shallow convex vase. Collectively these muscles are called the levator ani because that's what they do: elevate your anus, vagina, and bladder to keep them from falling through the bony pelvis and hitting the floor.

The levator ani muscles consist of the actual levator ani as well as the puborectalis, pubococcygeus, and ileococcygeus muscles. Forget these names. The only thing I want you to remember now is your ***perineum***. Your perineum is the area between the vaginal opening and the anus. The perineum is traversed by two of the pelvic floor muscles: the pubococcygeus and puborectalis. If you tear or have an episiotomy, these muscles are involved. These are not the anal sphincter muscles, but they do help provide continence (control over passing gas and bowel movements).

In repairing a tear or episiotomy your ob provider is re-approximating the torn ends of these muscles. It is crucial you have adequate anesthesia for your repair. If you don't it is difficult for your ob provider to do a good job. Communicate with her and tell her if you need more anesthetic for the repair.

Pregnancy by itself changes the anatomy of the pelvic floor. C-section does not prevent all these changes. More on this in the next chapter …

Many tears will be jagged and can be more challenging to repair than a straight cut, an episiotomy. A spontaneous tear usually causes less damage to the pelvic floor than an episiotomy. However, episiotomies still have a very important role in delivery.

Episiotomy

Episiotomy is a cut made in the perineum through the vaginal and perineal skin, and the puborectalis and pubococcygeus muscles. It is now undertaken with more consideration and gravity because a great body of research has shown cutting an episiotomy increases a woman's chances of having extension of that episiotomy to a third or fourth degree tear.

Most ob providers now take the approach that an episiotomy is just like any other surgery and must have an indication or medical reason to do one.

There are medical indications for episiotomies and you should trust your ob provider if she deems one is necessary for the safe delivery of your baby. Indications for episiotomy can include but are not limited to a severe drop in the fetal heart rate, necessitating expeditious delivery; delivery from the occiput posterior position, or to assist delivery with forceps or vacuum.

"Shredding"

Sometimes your ob provider may anticipate the delivery "shredding" your vagina and perineum, rather than producing a simple tear. This is rare and the "unofficial medical terminology" for

> **Trust your ob provider if he recommends cutting an episiotomy to avoid "shredding".**

it is "hamburger meat". If your ob provider anticipates you may have a complex, multi-pronged tear, or "shredded" perineum, she may cut an episiotomy to improve your chances of healing without future rectal and bladder dysfunction. A shredded perineum "explodes" the anatomy, requires many stitches, causes excess blood loss, and heals poorly. It is likely to need surgical revision six to twelve weeks post-partum. In some circumstances it can cause a tract to form between the rectum and vagina called a rectovaginal fistula. This results in stool coming out the vagina with no control and needs surgical repair.

If you say to your ob provider "Under no circumstances do I want an episiotomy," you may be saying "yes" to a shredded vagina.

Trust your ob provider. If he recommends an episiotomy to avoid "shredding", agree to it. You will save yourself and him a mountain of pain and aggravation and the possible necessity of a later operation under anesthesia to correct the damage sustained in "shredding".

Caput Succedaneum: Funny Looking Head

Your baby's skull is not one great big sphere of bone. Rather it is composed of several concave bones joined by cartilaginous "sutures". This allows for "molding" of the head so it can elongate and fit through the birth canal. By the time the baby is born the head will be elliptical rather than round and will have swelling at the crown called "caput succedaneum". This swelling is normal and is due to edema or fluid trapped in the scalp skin by the pressure of the pelvis on the baby's head. Your baby's head will assume a more rounded "cute" shape over the next twenty-four hours. However, just after birth most babies have "funny looking heads", and are not necessarily "cute". This is what the hat is for. Oh—and to keep the baby warm.

If your baby was delivered with assistance of forceps or vacuum there may be some additional swelling or bruising. This is all temporary and resolves within the first two days of life.

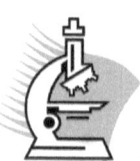

Science Notes: Baby's First Breaths

During the first few seconds of life the baby transforms from an inhabitant of water to an inhabitant of air. The idea that the baby's lungs begin as collapsed organs that "inflate" with air is a misconception. The lung sacs (alveoli) are already distended *in utero* by amniotic fluid. Rather than being "inflated" the air sacs are drained of fluid by a process that involves opening of microscopic "pores" between the lung sacs and the baby's lung capillaries which results in absorption of the lung fluid into the circulation.

With the first few breaths a chemical called surfactant coats the inside of the alveoli to reduce the surface tension or electric attraction between water molecules and help the baby keep her lung sacs inflated. Surfactant resembles soap. It is often lacking in the lungs of premature babies and its absence can produce "respiratory distress" in which the surface tension is too high between the water molecules in the baby's lungs, resulting in a collapse of the alveoli and inability to maintain lung inflation. Fortunately synthetic surfactant is available and has revolutionized the treatment of premature babies.

Seconds after the first breath fluid exits the baby's lungs and is replaced by air. As the fluid is replaced by air, the external pressure on the baby's lung capillaries decreases and circulation improves. By the fifth breath the baby's lungs are functioning similar to those of an adult with respect to their pressure-volume relationships and exchange of air.

Delivery of the Placenta: Third Stage

Just when you thought you were done, you may feel a gush of fluid from your vagina accompanied by contractions and the urge to push. This is the placenta. It normally separates within

> **Third Stage = Delivery of baby to delivery of placenta.**

thirty minutes of birth. One of the layers attaching the placenta to the uterus is a sheet of collagenous connective tissue called "Nitabuch's layer" after the man who discovered it. This layer splits and allows your placenta to shear away from the uterus.

After the placenta delivers your uterus shrinks to about twenty percent of its pregnancy size. With contraction of the uterine muscle fibers, the muscle fibers encircle the vessels and clamp them off, thereby minimizing blood loss.

It is crucial third stage is managed appropriately to prevent you from hemorrhaging and requiring a blood transfusion. The main techniques for the management of third stage are "fundal massage" and infusion of a dilute solution of oxytocin (Pitocin) after the placenta has delivered.

Fundal massage involves a nurse compressing the top of your uterus by deeply massaging your navel area in a circular fashion. It is not comfortable but necessary. You could do the same thing yourself but you are unlikely to exert adequate pressure to produce essential contraction of the uterine muscle because, well, it *hurts*. And the last thing you want after pushing a bowling ball through your bottom is for someone to mash on your tummy. Many apologies but it's important.

It is standard of care in the United States to infuse a dilute solution of oxytocin after the placenta has delivered. This practice reduces your blood loss and minimizes or prevents you from needing a blood transfusion. You can refuse this but there is sound medical science behind the practice.

Your baby's delivered, the placenta is out. Congratulations, you're ready for the "fourth trimester: Establishing lactation and the baby's first three months of life.

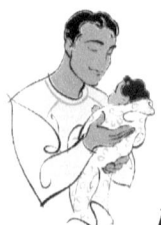

For Dads

"Shock," is the first word my husband used to describe the birth of our son. Mind you my husband possessed the "advantage" of absorbing all this obstetric knowledge by osmosis, merely by being my spouse.

"What do you mean, *shock*?" I demanded, "Did you think he wasn't *cute*—were you put off by the gory mess—were you distracted by the whole bottom thing and how sex would change—what do you mean SHOCK!!?" (All this in rapid fire manic wifely disbelief).

"No, none of that," he replied. "It's just that you had nine months feeling him inside you and getting used to him being there. For me it was like, there was his head and then boom! There *he* was, *all* of him. I suddenly realized this is real—here is this new person. I'd better grow up a little. Life has permanently changed and for the next eighteen years I'm responsible for making sure he turns out right."

Some guys are really into the birth thing—they're great coaches, very supportive. Others are a bit freaked out and anxious. Most are in-between. I've never actually seen a dad pass out but many have turned green and had to leave the room to "get some air."

My husband described the feeling as "All my senses were alive. I could see things more sharply, I heard things more clearly and my face felt red and hot."

"With the second one there wasn't any shock and I was able to enjoy the experience more," he said. "I knew she was coming and I was glad when she was finally here."

How a dad reacts to labor and birth is specific, momentary, and visceral. It does not necessarily portend what kind of a father he'll be.

Office Notes:

The Ten Page, Single-Spaced, Highlighted in Red Birth Plan

A week before her due date Mrs. Smith came to the office for a check-up and thrust at me a document, "Here. This is my Birth Plan."

I was used to receiving these, so at first I wasn't fazed. Until I delved into it. Mrs. Smith had culled it from the Internet, her birth classes, pregnancy books, friends, relatives and other sources—she seemed to have developed a reactionary paragraph to every pregnancy nightmare. In addition to the usual "I want the baby to nurse immediately," and "I want dad to cut the cord," it contained sentences like, "I want a COMPLETELY NATURAL CHILDBIRTH (in red caps) Do NOT give me ANY pain medication EVEN IF I'M BEGGING FOR IT." And "I ABSOLUTELY DO NOT want to have A VACUUM, FORCEPS OR C-SECTION." (Again—all this in red, as if by putting it in red caps I can wave a magic wand and have her birth go *perfectly*.) "And by NO MEANS will you give me an EPISIOTOMY!"

Well. After reading it I looked up at her and, shaking my head, said, "We'll do our best, but we only have so much control over labor," (to impart the understanding it's not *all* under *my* control). Mrs. Smith narrowed her eyes and fixed them on me like she was vaporizing the She-Devil.

I knew she was doomed.

Mrs. Smith pushed for four hours. She screamed and clawed at her husband until the poor guy looked like he'd had an unfortunate encounter with a rabid cat. Her baby was asynclitic and I felt part of that was due to her being very tense with all her pelvic muscles "bound up". After the fourth hour of pushing she finally consented to an epidural. Despite receiving it, she was still unable to deliver because her bottom was swollen and the baby's head was still tilted. I explained I would need to help her out with a vacuum.

At hour five she consented to the vacuum but said, "I absolutely DO NOT WANT AN EPISIOTOMY!"

"I'm concerned you might have a jagged tear, which might heal poorly."

Again she fixed me with the She-Devil gaze. So I didn't cut an episiotomy for fear she'd chop off my hand.

By this time the baby was showing signs of heart rate abnormalities from labor fatigue. I performed a vacuum delivery for a healthy but tired baby (and mom).

Mrs. Smith's bottom exploded. It took me an hour to repair (piecing together unrecognizable fragments of muscle and vagina); and I still had to bring her back to the operating room six weeks post-partum to revise a non-healing perineum.

For her next pregnancy Mrs. Smith's Birth Plan was a mere seven pages. She wanted a C-section.

Chapter 7

Help is on Its Way—Medical Intervention at Term and During Birth

Delivery is Usually Uneventful: The Big Picture

Two thirds of you will have normal uncomplicated vaginal births. This doesn't mean it will be easy or fast. For some of you, it will—labor will hit like a freight train and **boom**, an hour later, there's baby—especially if this is not your first. For others, you will endure a twenty-four hour labor but will have a vaginal birth at the end. Most will fall in-between.

However, all babies must come out one way or another and some of you will need assistance to have a healthy mom and healthy baby. In the United States the primary cesarean section rate for head-down (vertex) babies at most hospitals ranges from five to fifteen percent. This varies depending on the average level of medical risk patient the hospital handles. For example, teaching institutions and large inner-city hospitals with a neonatal intensive care unit handle a higher level of risk client as they are often referred complicated patients from other institutions. Therefore, their cesarean section rates may differ from community hospitals or hospitals lacking a neonatal intensive care unit.

About five percent of you will have vacuum or forceps-assisted vaginal deliveries.

> A "**primary cesarean section**" is a first cesarean section. A "**repeat cesarean section**" is just that.

These interventions are usually conducted for a prolonged second stage due to the baby's size, position, or maternal exhaustion.

The most common reasons to perform a primary C-section during term labor are arrest of dilation and arrest of descent. These are when the cervix fails to dilate and the baby fails to move down the birth canal. The ultimate causes of these dysfunctions of labor are: baby is too large to fit through pelvis; pelvis is too narrow; or baby is in a difficult position for delivery (asynclitic, occiput posterior; other abnormal presentations such as face or brow). Less commonly a primary C-section during labor may be performed for an abnormal fetal heart rate signifying fetal intolerance to labor. This is not automatic: If vaginal delivery is about to occur, or can be assisted with forceps or vacuum it is often safer and more expedient to deliver a baby not tolerating labor vaginally with or without assistance. However, if you are "remote from delivery"—the cervix is not fully dilated and the anticipated time to delivery exceeds the time the baby can tolerate the abnormal heart rate—a C-section will be performed for fetal safety.

Chapter Disclaimer: The Gory Details

The remainder of this chapter details medical interventions—the whys, whereas, and hows, undertaken when complications arise. Some women thrive on the gory details; others are nauseated. If it's too much information for you, no sweat—skip to the next chapter. Otherwise … read on and learn. Knowledge is power.

The National Cesarean Section Rate

You've probably seen in the media that the national C-section rate has risen in the last five years. Prior to 2000 the C-section rate was in decline from about thirty percent in the 1980's to about twenty percent at the turn of the century. The main reason for this drop was the practice of vaginal birth after cesarean section (VBAC). The increase in VBACs between the late 1970's to the late 1990's resulted in a decline in the overall C-section rate. However, due to liability considerations, since 2001 many hospitals no longer perform VBACs. The cessation of VBACs has caused the national C-section rate to rise again, so now it's approaching thirty percent.

Another factor behind the increasing C-section rate is a phenomenon known as "Patient Choice Cesarean Section". This movement started in South America in the 1990's, and has migrated to the United States. Because safety of cesarean section has become similar to that of vaginal birth, with declining rates of infection and blood transfusion, a few women now request a primary C-section without labor for a variety of reasons. Some have mothers or sisters who had "horrible birth experiences" and they don't want to repeat those experiences. Others are convinced it protects the pelvic floor and prevents urinary incontinence later in life. This is a partial myth and will be discussed in detail in the section entitled "Patient Choice Cesarean Section".

The Breech Position

Six to seven percent of singleton babies are breech—butt down—at thirty-seven weeks. Although babies can safely delivery from the breech position, this practice is disappearing, again due to safety and liability concerns. If your baby is breech at term you may be offered an external cephalic version—an attempt to turn the baby from the outside. The success rate for version is about fifty percent. If you decline a version, or have an unsuccessful one performed, your ob provider will most likely recommend a scheduled C-section at thirty-nine weeks for delivery.

Vaginal delivery of a breech is safe if five conditions are met: your pelvis is roomy; the baby is full term and of average size; the baby's head is flexed; and the baby is in the "frank breech" position with hips flexed and legs extended at the knees. You will probably be offered a vaginal breech delivery only if your ob provider is an "old-timer" with nerves of steel or you deliver at a teaching institution. Even though many obstetricians are still trained in vaginal breech delivery, most of them don't want to deal with the medical-legal risk so they won't offer the vaginal breech option to their clients. As fewer obstetricians regularly perform vaginal breech delivery, competency will decline and the option will vanish altogether.

The rationale for the above five conditions is to avoid "head entrapment". Head entrapment can occur with a breech delivery because the softer body of the baby may not dilate the cervix enough to allow the hard head to pass through. It can by complicated by the head being too extended to fit through the birth canal. Head entrapment is a rare but dangerous condition that can pose a risk for fetal death or paralysis.

Breech delivery of a second twin

Breech delivery of a second twin is an entirely different matter than breech delivery of a singleton fetus. With twins, if the first baby is in the vertex position, it is extremely safe to deliver the second twin vaginally by "breech extraction".

> **Breech Extraction of a second twin is as safe, and more expedient, than C-section for a second twin.**

For obstetricians trained and experienced in this technique vaginal delivery of a second twin is as safe, and more expedient, than C-section for a breech second twin.

With twins the first baby fully dilates the cervix as long as he is head-down. Thus, the risk for head entrapment of a second twin is near non-existent. The only caveat to this is if the head of the breech second twin is hyper-extended, or "star-gazing". If your ob provider offers you vaginal delivery for a breech second twin, she will check the twin's position and size with the ultrasound before attempting it.

Breech extraction is one of the most fun deliveries for an obstetrician because it's safe, easy and saves the mother from having a C-section. After confirming the second twin remains in the breech position and the head is flexed, she grasps the feet of the second twin and gently pulls the baby out by the feet. When the baby has delivered to the shoulder blades, an assistant supports the baby while the obstetrician rotates the baby clockwise and counter-clockwise to deliver each arm. She then presses on the baby's chin to keep the head flexed and delivers the head. It looks like magic but usually the breech second twin practically "falls out" after the initial extraction of the feet and lower body.

Induction of Labor

Labor is induced for a multitude of reasons: sometimes for the health of the mother (such as with pre-eclampsia), other times for the health of the fetus (such as with poor fetal growth or overdue fetus); and at times electively or for the convenience of the mother or physician.

The method of induction depends on the status of your cervix and the reason for induction. If your cervix is thick and closed it is considered "unfavorable" for induction. If it is already dilated and thinned it is considered "favorable". In the case of the former, induction is initiated with prostaglandins; for the latter—pitocin (oxytocin) is used.

Some Reasons for Labor Inductions

Maternal	Fetal
Pre-eclampsia	Medical or obstetric complications that jeopardize fetal well being
Diabetes	Poor Fetal Growth
Rupture of membranes without labor	Rupture of membranes without labor
Other obstetric or medical complications	Post-dates (overdue)
Elective (e.g. TOBP—"Tired of Being Pregnant")	

Prostaglandins Ripen the Unfavorable Cervix

Natural prostaglandins are involved in the commencement of normal labor. Pharmaceutical preparations (misoprostol—Cytotec, Prepidil, and Cervidil) are used to soften and thin ("ripen") an unfavorable cervix. Prostaglandins are placed vaginally and they result in a reorganization of the collagen (connective tissue) of the cervix, and an increase in the fluid content of the cervix. This shortens and softens the cervix.

Often vaginal prostaglandins initiate labor in addition to softening the cervix. When labor is induced with vaginal prostaglandins, it decreases the incidence of needing intravenous oxytocin and it shortens the interval between induction and delivery, compared to the use of intravenous oxytocin without prostaglandins.

> **Vaginal prostaglandins soften and shorten the cervix, and usually produce the onset of labor.**

Augmentation of Labor with Amniotomy (Breaking the Water)

Breaking the water is done with a plastic "amnio hook". It is not painful. The birth attendant inserts the amnio hook and passes it along her finger to guide it to the bag of waters. The hook can be used to open the bag. Breaking the water (amniotomy) stimulates contractions to come more frequently and with greater force. It can jump start a stalled-out labor.

Amniotomy also allows for the hard fetal head to push directly against the cervix, rather than the buoyant fluid-filled amniotic sac. This increases the ability of the uterus to dilate the cervix.

In the picture below, a balloon is inflated to simulate the bag of waters. The amnio hook is the device in the left side of the picture, indenting the balloon.

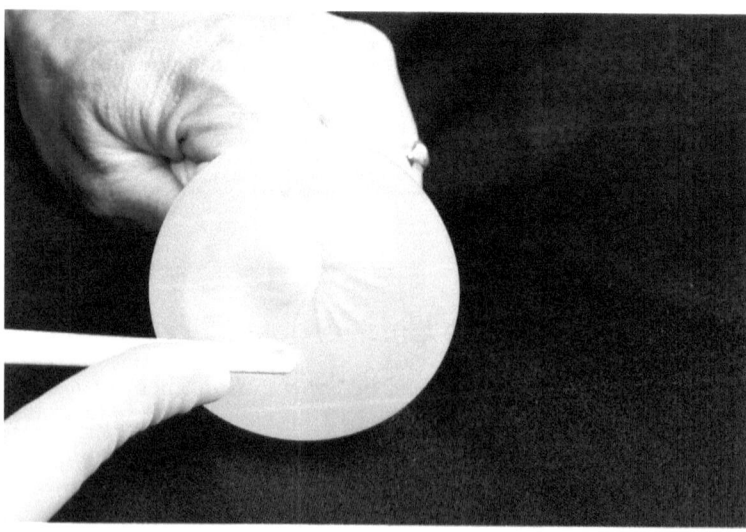

Induction of Labor with Oxytocin (Pitocin)

If your cervix is short, soft, and dilated induction may begin with oxytocin (pitocin). This is an intravenous infusion of a synthetic version of the hormone, oxytocin, normally made by

> **Lack of Dilation: Cervix stops or fails to dilate.**

the brain. Oxytocin increases the strength, frequency, and duration of your contractions. An oxytocin-induced labor differs from one induced with prostaglandins because it feels like flicking a switch and having contractions. There is no gradual build-up, as with prostaglandins. However, in certain circumstances (as with a dilated cervix) oxytocin may be more effective at bringing on labor than prostaglandins.

Augmentation of labor with oxytocin

> **Lack of Descent: Baby fails to move down the birth canal.**

Oxytocin is use more frequently to *augment* rather than initiate labor. The goal of augmentation is to assist with or correct a dysfunctional labor to allow for safe vaginal delivery.

Labor dysfunction

Labor dysfunction comes in two varieties: lack of dilation and lack of descent of the fetal head. Often they coexist to add up to: the baby's not moving down the pelvis. The ultimate underlying causes of dysfunctional labor are many but can be distilled to problems with power, passenger, and pelvis.

Table 8.2 Causes of Dysfunctional Labor: Power, Passenger, Pelvis

Power = Uterus And Maternal Pushing	Passenger = Fetus	Pelvis = Maternal factors
Uterus stops contracting—uterine fatigue.	Fetus too big for pelvis	Pelvic inlet too narrow
Uterus contracts infrequently (uterine fatigue)	Fetus in poor position for vaginal delivery (asynclitic, occiput posterior)	Pelvic outlet too narrow (pubic arch)
Uterus contracts but weakly (uterine fatigue)	Fetus not tolerating labor	Soft tissue swelling from long labor
Mother is exhausted and unable to push effectively	Large fetus exacerbates maternal exhaustion	Maternal obesity limits room in pelvis

Increasing the frequency, force and duration of contractions with oxytocin can ameliorate many of these dysfunctions of labor to allow successful vaginal birth.

Other Reasons for Intervention

Fetal Intolerance of Labor

Normal and abnormal fetal heart rates were defined in the previous chapter. Abnormal fetal heart rates result from one of two major causes: cord compression and placental insufficiency. All measures to resuscitate or improve fetal status *in utero* are directed at improving blood flow to the placenta, relieving cord compression, and increasing maternal blood oxygen concentration to improve the oxygenation of the blood traveling to the fetus.

Relief of Cord Compression

Maternal position change—usually lying on the left side or getting on hands and knees—displaces the weight of the uterus off the aorta and inferior vena cava. These are the major vessels circulating blood to the uterus, placenta, and fetus. Moving the weight of the uterus off these pipelines can increase blood flow enough to relieve stress to the fetus. Changes in maternal position can also provide relief from cord compression by effecting a change in fetal position to reduce the cord compression. These measures can normalize the fetal heart rate and provide the baby with enough reserve to complete labor.

It is common for the cord to be compressed intermittently during labor, mostly during second stage as the baby is moving through the vagina. These episodes are usually quick followed by rapid recovery of the fetus. Brief intervals of cord compression do not produce any short-term or long-term ill effects on the baby.

In some situations such as cord prolapse, your obstetric provider may physically manipulate the baby's head in an attempt to reduce the compression of the cord. Cord prolapse occurs when the umbilical cord slips through the cervix before the head and precedes the head. It is rare but if it's going to happen it often occurs as the membranes rupture if the head is not well applied to the cervix. Sometimes the head can be adjusted and the cord prolapse reduced. If this is not possible and cord compression or prolapse compromises fetal status, a cesarean delivery will be performed.

Relief of Placental Insufficiency: Terbutaline

If the fetal status is aggravated by the frequency and intensity of uterine contractions placental insufficiency may be the culprit. In addition to maternal position change and oxygen administration another technique may be employed to relieve placental insufficiency.

Terbutaline is a medication that relaxes the uterus and may cause cessation of contractions. Terbutaline is used to treat preterm labor (see Chapter Four); but at term it is employed for intrauterine resuscitation. By decreasing or stopping contractions, the uterus relaxes; the blood vessels endure less compression and blood supply to the placenta and fetus improves.

Placental insufficiency may be caused by an aging placenta (being overdue), maternal hypertension and other medical conditions, smoking, and drug use such as cocaine or amphetamines. Sometimes the placenta simply implants abnormally; and poor placental architecture causes insufficiency with the stress of labor contractions.

At other times these measures are unsuccessful and on occasion call for an emergency cesarean delivery if the cervix is not fully dilated; or an assisted vaginal delivery if the cervix is dilated.

Shoulder dystocia

Shoulder dystocia is defined as delivery of the head with subsequent entrapment of the baby's front (anterior) shoulder behind the pubic bone. Large babies, maternal gestational diabetes, and maternal obesity are risk factors for shoulder dystocia. However, the majority of shoulder dystocia is unexpected and occurs with normal size babies in average size women.

Anticipation and use of momentum are crucial

> **Measures to combat shoulder dystocia:**
> 1) **McRobert's maneuver**
> 2) **Suprapubic pressure**
> 3) **"Wood's corkscrew" and delivery of the posterior arm**
> 4) **Cutting a large episiotomy or even third- or fourth-degree opening**
> 5) **Intentional fracture of the fetal clavicle (collar bone)**
> 6) **Zavanelli maneuver (replacing the fetal head into the pelvis and performing Cesearean section**
> 7) **Symphysisotomy—cutting the pubic symphysis cartilage to release the impacted shoulder.**

to managing suspected shoulder dystocia. If your ob provider is concerned the shoulders may get stuck, she'll often have you continue pushing until the front shoulder is out, before stopping to suction out the nose and mouth. This makes use of the forward momentum and prevents "backsliding" or sucking of the head against the perineum and further impacting the shoulder under the pubic bone.

If it can't be prevented, several maneuvers are undertaken to reduce shoulder dystocia and complete vaginal birth. Your participation in these maneuvers is essential and can make the difference between safe vaginal birth and disaster. The first two of these are usually employed together; while the final two are "last resorts".

The **McRobert's maneuver** is an "Ultra C" position (see Chapter Six) in which you're asked to draw your knees up to your chest and out as far as possible in order to rotate the pubic bone over the entrapped shoulder.

The second maneuver is **suprapubic pressure** in which a birth assistant applies pressure with her palm above your pubic bone to dislodge the impacted shoulder. Together McRobert's maneuver and suprapubic pressure reduce the majority of shoulder dystocias; and no further maneuvers are required.

Failing this, the third maneuver, **"Wood's corkscrew"** involves your birth attendant manually rotating the posterior shoulder forward in an attempt to position the baby in the longer diagonal axis of the pelvic outlet rather than the shorter front-to-back axis. This is often accompanied by **delivery of the posterior arm** in which the provider grasps the baby's arm closest to the floor and rotates it across the baby's chest to deliver that arm—the impacted shoulder usually follows.

If this fails the provider may intentionally **fracture one of the clavicles** (collar bone) to create a smaller diameter for delivery. This is done by pulling outward on the clavicle—it does not disrupt any vessels or nerves and reduces the chances of permanent nerve damage to the impacted arm. Fracture of the neonatal clavicle can occur in normal vaginal birth and be unrecognized. Intentional or not, they heal quickly and rarely cause permanent problems.

Last ditch efforts are **cutting a large episiotomy** ("vaginal C-section"), **cutting the pubic symphysis**, or replacing the fetal head in the vagina and performing a Cesarean section (**Zavanelli maneuver**).

Assisted Vaginal Delivery

Sometime babies just don't come out without help. There are many medical indications for assisted vaginal delivery and this is a safe way to have your baby. The most common reasons for performing a vacuum or forceps delivery are arrest of second stage (baby stuck while pushing), fetal intolerance of second stage, maternal exhaustion, and fetal malposition such as occiput posterior or asynclitism.

All babies must come out one way or another. So if you're baby's not coming keep in mind, if you say "Absolutely No," to vacuum or forceps, you will be saying "Yes," to cesarean section.

As with any surgery there are risks and benefits. Usually the benefits of a forceps or vacuum outweigh the risks, as long as safety criteria are met.

Safety Requirements for Vacuum/Forceps

Safety criteria for either a vacuum or forceps delivery are the same: The cervix must be fully dilated. The largest diameter of the head must be at the mid-pelvis—that means the leading edge of the head is well into the vaginal canal, past the majority of the bony pelvis. The rotation of the head must be less than forty-five degrees off the midline.

If the head is directly facing mom's side and the baby's not moving down the birth canal, this is a condition called **deep transverse arrest**. Often this baby cannot deliver vaginally because too much rotation would be required with vacuum or forceps to be performed safely.

The operator must know the position and degree of descent of the head and be well trained in the performance of vacuum or forceps deliveries. The operator must also be willing to abandon the attempt if it's unsuccessful after a reasonable amount of tries.

If your baby needs assisted vaginal delivery your ob provider will discuss the reasons why. You always have the option to refuse but you may be trading a safe assisted vaginal delivery for a cesarean section.

In certain situations such as a low fetal heart rate, a forceps or vacuum delivery may be the safest and fastest route of delivery. Your baby may not tolerate the time required to move you to the operating room and prepare for a cesarean. A forceps or vacuum can have a baby delivered in minutes.

Vacuum

Depending on your geographic area, vacuum deliveries comprise five to ten percent of all vaginal deliveries. Vacuum delivery is safe when done according to established standards. The vacuum is a flexible cup applied to the fetal head. Vacuum is applied with a hand pump to generate a specified amount of suction that is monitored on the vacuum device (400–500 mm Hg equal to 0.6 kg/cm^2 force on the fetal head). Gentle traction is exerted by the operator while mom pushes.

The vacuum does not increase risk to the baby when done properly. It should be applied to the midline and crown of the head, roughly equidistant between the front and rear soft spots or fontanelles. If the cup is applied too far forward on the head, it can exacerbate fetal neck extension and be of no help effecting delivery.

The operator should not "rock" the vacuum back and forth while exerting traction. If the head does not descend with normal vacuum pressure and traction, the vacuum should be abandoned and either forceps or cesarean should be performed. A "popoff" is a sign the vacuum isn't working. A "popoff" occurs when the cup unintentionally disengages from the head during traction. It is *not* synonymous with the operator intentionally releasing the vacuum pressure between pulls. Normally the operator *will* release the vacuum pressure between pulls to minimize the amount of time vacuum pressure is applied to the head. Generally three "popoffs" are considered acceptable before the method is abandoned.

Extended vacuum time (more than five minutes of applied vacuum) and excessive "popoffs" (more than three) is associated with an increased incidence of fetal cephalohematoma (bleeding under the scalp) and intracranial hemorrhage (bleeding inside the head). However, as long as the standards for use of vacuum are not exceeded, this is a safe method of delivery.

Forceps

Depending on your geographic area and place of delivery, forceps may account for three to eight percent of all vaginal deliveries.

Forceps deliveries are safe and are a thing of beauty when performed by an experienced practitioner. As with any medical procedure there are trade-offs. Many studies have shown forceps may increase the risk of vaginal tearing, but they have a lower incidence of injury to the baby such as cephalohematoma and shoulder dystocia compared to vacuum.

My experience as an obstetrician over the past fifteen years (confirmed by research) is that forceps result in decreased injury to the baby—cephalohematomas and intracranial bleeds.

While forceps may produce a slightly higher incidence of vaginal tears, the vacuum has a higher risk of vaginal "shredding". I find it much easier to repair a laceration than deal with "shredding". "Shredding" results in greater blood loss and is more difficult to repair because there is a broad abrasion rather than a defined laceration that can be closed with sutures. Sometimes the only solution to shredding is to place a pressure pack in the vagina and hope it heals—obviously not ideal for the mother or practitioner. Over time I have come to distrust vacuum and use forceps preferentially for (in my hands) their reduced incidence of causing fetal head bleeds and vaginal "shredding". Different practitioners develop different preferences and there is no one "right" way to do things as long as the operator adheres to national safety guidelines.

Forceps do not compress the head; rather they act like cupped hands that grip the head at its widest diameter and cradle it towards the chin. They provide a more accurate hold of the head, and thus greater control, than vacuum. Forceps are especially helpful delivering babies from the occiput posterior position. Forceps also allow for mild rotation (less than forty-five degrees) of the head to provide greater flexion and facilitate delivery. Forceps may leave slight bruises on the baby but these are temporary and usually gone by twenty-four hours of age.

If the baby can't be delivered vaginally through your own efforts, or with the assistance of forceps or vacuum, a cesarean delivery will be performed.

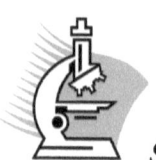

Science Notes: Forceps versus Vacuum Delivery

One of the largest recent studies done comparing forceps to vacuum delivery was conducted at the University of California, San Francisco, and published in 2005. It compared roughly 2000 forceps with 2000 vacuum deliveries.

In regards to fetal trauma: The rate of cephalohematoma with forceps was 4.5 % versus 14.8 % with vacuum. In other words, vacuum had a three-fold increase in the rate of fetal cephalohematoma. Shoulder dystocia was also more than doubled in the vacuum group (3.5%) versus forceps group (1.5%).

In this study maternal trauma was higher than in the forceps group – the rate of third and fourth degree perineal lacerations was 36.9% in the forceps group versus 26.8% in the vacuum group.

Vacuum and Forceps Delivery

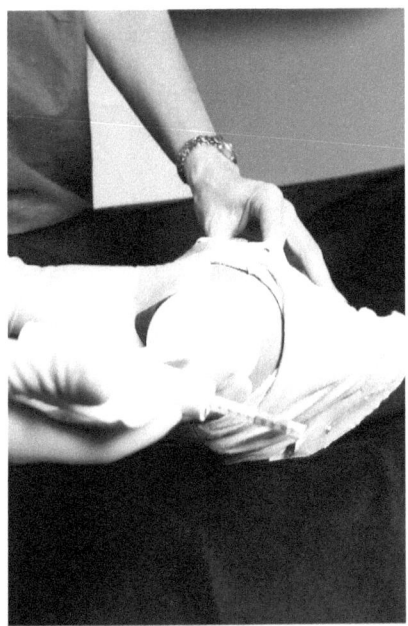

Left: Vacuum Application. Once the device is applied to the fetal head, the suction handle is pumped to 400 mm Hg (on right, slightly out of focus). The birth attendant exerts gentle downward and outward traction to deliver the head.

Right: Forceps application. The birth attendant introduces one blade at a time. The blade is introduced and positioned with the vaginal hand, not the top hand. The top hand merely supports the handle.

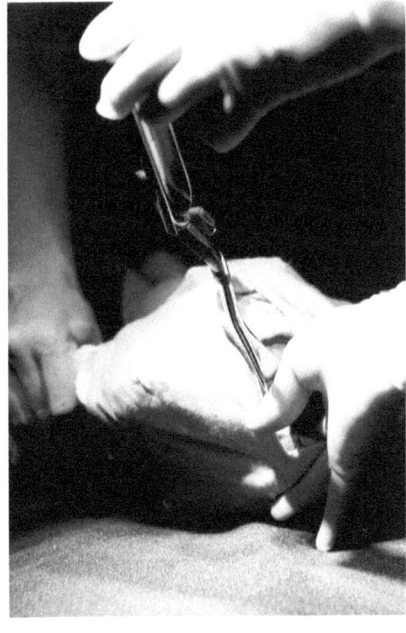

Vacuum and Forceps Delivery, continued ...

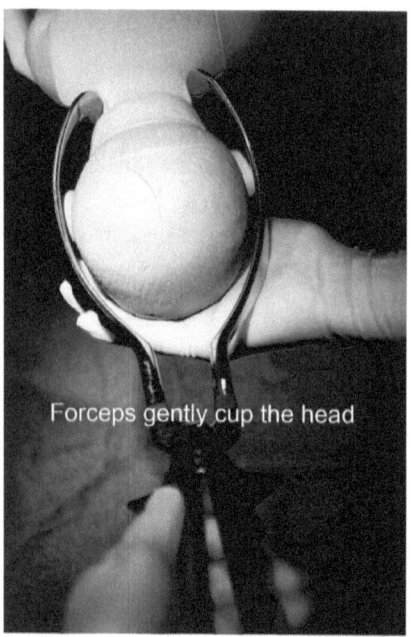

Forceps gently cup the head

Left: Forceps gently cup the head. They do not exert undue pressure when properly applied and positioned.

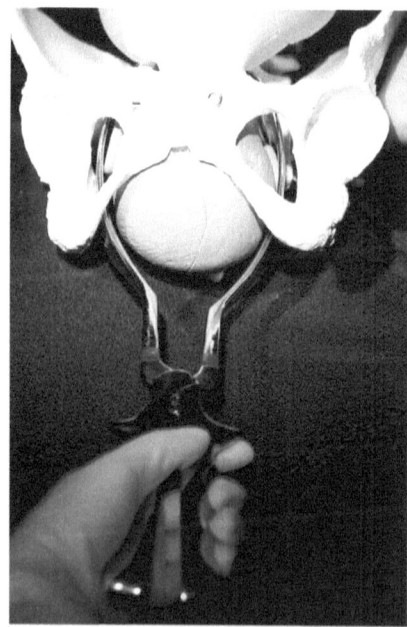

Right: Forceps applied to head in pelvis. The birth attendant exerts gentle traction downward and outward, following the axis of the vagina, to deliver the baby.

Cesarean Section

As stated above, Cesarean deliveries now account for about thirty percent of all births. Many of these are elective repeat C-sections due to many hospitals choosing to not offer VBAC (vaginal birth after cesarean).

The rate of primary cesarean (first C-section) is important in assessing a hospital or practitioner. It varies between five and twenty percent depending on the geographic region and the level of risk patient with which the hospital contends. For example, an inner-city referral hospital may do a large number of C-sections for high risk patients that are referred from other hospitals.

Primary C-sections are done for many indications, including breech, failure of the cervix to dilate or the head to descend in the pelvis, non-reassuring fetal heart rate patterns, and other less common issues of maternal and fetal health.

There are things you can do to minimize your risk of a cesarean. Throughout pregnancy watch your weight gain and stick to the guidelines given in Chapter One. Maternal obesity (body mass index over thirty) increases the risk of C-section three-to four-fold. This is thought to be due to larger babies and impedance of labor by maternal tissues.

Avoid tobacco and drugs such as cocaine and methamphetamines to minimize the risks of prematurity and placental abruption (see Chapter Four).

Walking in early labor has *not* been shown to decrease the rate of C-sections but it is helpful if for no other reason than it gives you something to do besides focus on your contractions. Besides, it can't hurt to make use of gravity as much as possible in early labor.

During pushing, make the most of your pushes using the tips given in Chapter Six on labor. Maintaining your C-position and keeping hips flexed keep the baby's head flexed and maximize the room in your pelvis.

Despite your and your practitioner's best efforts, it may prove to be impossible for you to deliver vaginally. This is not a failure on anyone's part, but a simple fact of life. Sometimes it's essential or safer to perform a cesarean section.

If you have a C-section it will usually be done under a regional (spinal or epidural) anesthetic so you're awake but numb from the waist down. This minimizes the amount of anesthetic exposure to the baby and allows you to be conscious to enjoy the birth of your baby. The difference between a labor epidural and a surgical epidural is the density of the block or amount and kind of anesthetic infused into the epidural catheter.

In some instances such as an extreme emergency (**rare**) or failure to obtain good anesthesia with a regional block, a general anesthetic will be performed.

If you go to C-section expect commotion. You'll be moved to an operating room. The room will fill with a cadre of medical personnel: In addition to your practitioner and labor nurse, there will be an anesthesiologist, a scrub nurse to hand your surgeon instruments, a surgical assistant to help hold retractors and cut suture, a circulating nurse to fetch supplies during surgery, a pediatrician, and a nurse for the baby. If you were laboring with a certified nurse midwife, she will often be the surgeon's assistant.

Once you have adequate anesthesia your spouse or support person will be allowed to enter the operating room. Most anesthesiologists will wait until you have a good anesthetic established before allowing your significant person into the operating room. Usually only one family member or support person is permitted due to the number of people already present, the size of the room, and the efficiency of the surgical team (they don't want to be tripping over a number of your family members).

After anesthesia is established, your abdomen is scrubbed with sterile solution; a catheter (tube) is inserted into the bladder to keep it drained during surgery. The bladder is located directly in front of the uterus and if it's too full, it can obstruct the surgeon's view and progress to the uterus. You won't feel the catheter insertion if it's done after your anesthetic is established. After surgery the catheter is removed the following morning or as soon as you're able to walk to the bathroom. To enhance sterility the operative site will be draped so as to allow only the site for surgery to be exposed.

A horizontal skin incision is made one to two inches above your pubic bone. The fat and fascia (connective tissue) underneath is opened and the abdominal muscles (rectus) are *spread apart*, not cut. The bladder is displaced downward from the uterus and the uterus is opened. The baby is brought up into the incision and delivered. Typical skin-to-baby time is one to two minutes. Exceptions to this are if you've had previous C-sections and have a lot of scar tissue.

Once the baby is delivered she's shown to you, handed to the pediatrician, and taken to the nursery while your surgery is completed. Your spouse or family member will accompany the baby, the pediatrician and baby nurse to the nursery while you're still in the operating room.

With the baby out, the placenta is removed from the uterus, the uterine incision is closed and all other tissue layers are re-joined with suture.

In rare instances the abdominal muscles may be cut during the course of a C-section in order to deliver the baby—this usually only occurs if you've had multiple previous C-sections with accumulation of scar tissue so as to not allow enough manual separation and relaxation of the abdominal muscles. If your abdominal muscles are cut they will heal by adhering to the overlying fascia. Realigning the fascia edges rejoins the muscles and eventually the muscle fibers intertwine to recreate a normal abdominal wall.

Total operative time for a C-section is usually fifteen to thirty minutes, barring extenuating circumstances such as extensive scar tissue, severe maternal obesity, or excessive bleeding during the procedure.

Once the surgery is complete you'll be moved to a post anesthesia care unit (PACU) or post op area. You'll remain there for about forty-five minutes for observation to ensure you're stable from the surgery. Some hospitals will allow your support person and baby to come back to the PACU to stay with you during this phase of recovery. Often your nurse will try to have you initiate lactation in the PACU as soon as you and the baby are ready.

What's dad doing while you're in the PACU? Well he's with the baby and the baby's nurse in the nursery. The pediatrician and baby nurse are checking the baby's medical status, weighing, and measuring him. Often dad will give baby his first bath at this time. The baby's nurse may be doing you a great favor and showing dad not only how to wash a baby, but how to change his diaper and how to wrap the baby in a blanket. A good nurse will show dad how his participation is immediate and necessary; and how he can make mom's life much easier by doing these little tasks.

Recovery from a C-section

Recovery from a C-section versus a vaginal birth differs most in the first few days. Beyond that, it's pretty much the same and is actually *recovery from pregnancy*, rather than the mode of delivery. Therefore, the bulk of your recovery will be addressed in Chapter Nine.

The biggest difference in how you'll feel after a C-section versus a vaginal birth is you'll have an abdominal incision. On the other hand, you won't feel like a Mack truck has driven through your bottom and you won't have perineal pain. (Everything's a trade-off.) Incision pain is treated initially with intravenous pain meds. This is often delivered via a PCA or Patient Controlled Analgesia pump—an I.V. with a button connected to it so you can administer pain medication to yourself as needed. As soon as you're able to eat solid food (either the same day or day after) you'll be switched to oral pain medication. Incision pain usually subsides within one to three days, similar to perineal pain from healing of a laceration or episiotomy. This will be addressed more in the next chapter.

Having a C-section does not affect lactation or bonding. Most birth units will try to get you breastfeeding within an hour of delivery as long as you and the baby are medically stable.

Hospital stay after a C-section is usually two to four days versus one to two days for a vaginal birth.

VBAC versus Elective Repeat C-section

The practice of vaginal birth after C-section (VBAC) has see-sawed over the past thirty years. Prior to the 1980s the adage was "Once a Cesarean, Always a Cesarean," meaning once you had a C-

> **Consequences of uterine rupture range from asymptomatic to medical disaster.**

section all your future births would be via C-section. However, research showed that a vaginal "trial of labor" after one cesarean section was fairly safe. Therefore during the 1980's and early 1990's VBAC was increasingly offered to women as an option. During this era about seventy percent of eligible women had successful VBAC's. Most repeat C-sections done during a trial of labor for a VBAC are done for failure to progress in labor, rather than fetal or maternal compromise.

The risk of a VBAC is uterine rupture. After one previous C-section, the risk of uterine rupture is about 0.5 to one percent; after two previous C-sections, the risk of uterine rupture is roughly two percent. Agents to induce or augment labor, such as prostaglandins or oxytocin, can increase the risk of uterine rupture up to three to five percent.

Uterine rupture in itself isn't always a big deal—it can be repaired. Some uterine ruptures or "dehiscences" (separation of the uterus at the previous C-section site) are asymptomatic, and not diagnosed until after the baby is born and the practitioner examines the scar vaginally to discover the previous scar has separated. In this case, mom will be taken to surgery to repair the scar.

However, the consequences of uterine rupture can be disastrous and it can evolve into a dire medical emergency. If the uterus ruptures there is a high risk (thirty to fifty percent, depending on the study you read) of loss of blood supply to the baby causing serious neurologic injury or even fetal death.

For mom uterine rupture can extend to the uterine arteries, resulting in serious blood loss, transfusion, and even hysterectomy if the rupture can't be surgically repaired in a timely fashion.

So if VBAC's are usually "safe" and successful seventy percent of the time, what has happened to VBAC in the past ten years? To some extent there has been a rethinking of VBAC's among the medical community since a "definitive" study on the issue was published in the New England Journal of Medicine in 1999. However, the findings of that study were largely consistent with previous knowledge about VBAC's.

The practice of VBAC has declined over the past ten years due in part to rethinking VBAC's, but also to lawsuits and insurance companies. VBAC's gone awry have constituted some of the largest jury awards and losses for medical malpractice insurance companies. As a result, many medical malpractice companies place strict requirements (regarding in-house staff and anesthesia) on insuring hospitals and physicians doing VBAC's, or they simply won't insure providers to do VBAC's at all. Many small, rural, or community hospitals can't meet the in-house staffing requirements for VBAC's—twenty four hour in-house availability of the obstetrician, anesthesiologist, and an operating room crew. Thus, VBAC's have declined as an option in these settings.

Some practitioners simply don't want to deal with the headache of VBAC's. It requires they drop everything and hang around the hospital during your entire labor. This means if they had office patients, all of these are cancelled so your physician can be available in the hospital during your six or twelve or fifteen hour labor. The reimbursement for VBAC's does not adequately compensate the physician for her foregone office income and time spent in the hospital waiting for you to deliver.

However, VBAC remains an option at many teaching hospitals with 24-7 staffing by resident physicians, anesthesiologists, and operating room crews. Some larger non-teaching institutions offer VBAC's, as they have the resources to meet the staffing requirements. If your hospital doesn't offer VBAC's, and you desire one, if you're willing to travel, you're likely to find one that does.

Patient Choice Cesarean Section (PCCS)

What is patient choice Cesarean section? It's a movement that originated in the 1990s in South America in which women opt to have a cesarean section without labor, rather than go through labor. Why would women want this? Many reasons.

Avoiding vaginal birth prevents trauma to the vagina and perineum. It eliminates a great degree of the stretching of the vagina. A traumatic vaginal birth in which a woman sustains a laceration through the anal sphincter and rectum has been likened to a "vaginal C-section" in which the vagina has been opened nearly the length of a C-section incision. These complications of vaginal birth occur in fewer than five percent of deliveries but—ouch! The mere—albeit unlikely—possibility of having your bottom explode deters enough women from wanting to attempt vaginal birth that PCCS has migrated from South America and taken hold in our society.

The typical woman in the United States who requests PCCS is someone whose sister or mother had traumatic vaginal births with attempts at vacuum, forceps, and ultimately C-section. Also women with narrow pelvises and/or large babies frequently request PCCS. Some women have already had a traumatic vaginal birth and they don't want to repeat the experience so they request PCCS. There is also a small percent of women who are simply very nervous about labor and desire a PCCS.

As surgery has become safer with the advent of better sterile technique, antibiotics, and improved operative technique cesarean section is now viewed by many to be nearly as safe as vaginal birth. The risk of major complications such as transfusion, infection, and inadvertent surgical injury to other organs is less than one percent.

Some physicians are recommending PCCS for women with high risk medical or family histories or extreme anxiety about vaginal labor.

There is also an emerging philosophy among physicians and women that PCCS prevents later problems with urinary and fecal incontinence that can be precipitated by vaginal birth. Beware of this thinking. There is no definitive scientific proof that cesarean section prevents future incontinence and surgeries for this problem. In fact over the years I have performed hundreds of incontinence procedures for women who had only cesarean births.

Recent studies on the pelvic muscles and nerves have shown that twenty-five percent of the weakening of the pelvic floor muscles *occurs during pregnancy before labor*. The weight of the pregnancy stretches and damages the nerves that innervate the pelvic muscles. So just carrying a pregnancy to term affects pelvic floor muscles and nerves. Try not to be discouraged by this—do your Kegel exercises to give your pelvic floor the best chance to endure pregnancy and birth with as minimal damage as possible. (Kegels are discussed in detail in Chapters Six and Eight.)

Management of Third Stage (Delivery of the Placenta) and Postpartum Hemorrhage

The major causes of post-partum hemorrhage are three: Uterine atony, retained placenta, and lacerations. Average blood loss for a normal delivery is about 300-500 mL or one to two pints. Blood loss in excess of 500 mL defines post-partum hemorrhage. How do you know if you're having a post-partum hemorrhage? If you observe a look of concern on your birth attendant's face and you hear liquid dripping on the floor, you're having post-partum hemorrhage.

Uterine Atony

After expulsion of the placenta the uterus muscle contracts down around the vessels within the muscle wall. This constricts the vessels and minimizes blood loss.

If the uterus fails to contract down the vessels aren't crimped and excess bleeding can result. This is called uterine atony and literally occurs because the uterus muscle is tired. Uterine atony

> **"Audible blood loss is not a good thing."**

occurs most often after a long labor, delivery of a large baby, in women who've had many previous births ("grand multiparity"), or in the presence of intrauterine infection.

Uterine atony is treated with uterotonic agents—medications that stimulate the uterine muscle to contract. These include oxytocin, methergine, hemabate, and Cytotec. These medications are used sequentially in order of their side effects. However, Cytotec, given rectally in a dose of 800 micrograms is becoming more common as a first-line drug as it is as effective as the other drugs and it does not require an intravenous infusion or intramuscular injection (shot) to administer. There is a movement by the American College of Obstetrician-Gynecologists and other health organizations to distribute Cytotec free to communities, lay mid-wives, and "shamans" in third world countries such as Africa because postpartum hemorrhage is a leading cause of maternal death in these countries. Post-partum hemorrhage is treatable, and if managed correctly, saves a woman's life.

In U.S. hospitals it is standard practice to massage the uterus and infuse a dilute solution of oxytocin after the placenta is out to help the uterus clamp down and minimize your blood loss and risk of transfusion. Uterine massage (from the outside) stimulates your uterus muscle to contract and remain that way—you can massage your own uterus. Just ask your nurse to identify it for you and help you with proper technique.

Retained Placenta

A rarer cause of post-partum hemorrhage is retained placenta or amniotic membranes. Your provider will inspect the placenta after delivery to determine if it appears intact, or if sections are missing. The placenta normally delivers within forty-five minutes of the baby. Risk factors for retained placenta include history of previous placental separation (abruption), abnormal attachment of the placenta, chronic high blood pressure, or previous uterine surgery.

Sometimes the placenta fails altogether to separate and deliver spontaneously. In this situation a manual removal of the placenta will be performed, usually under "conscious sedation" if you do not have an epidural for anesthesia. Conscious sedation is light sedatives and anesthetics to allow you to sleep briefly through a procedure without needing respiratory support as you would with full anesthesia.

Medications given for conscious sedation, such as Versed and Fentanyl, are quick-acting, allow you to "sleep" for about ten minutes and easily reversible.

A manual removal of the placenta involves the provider inserting her hand in the uterus and manipulating the placenta away from the uterine interior. When a manual removal is performed it is often accompanied by curettage, or scraping of the uterine wall to rid it of any fragments of membranes and placenta. Manual removals and curettage can be done in the LDR or in the operating room, depending on the medical situation and set-up at your place of delivery.

Retained placenta and membranes is not always diagnosed at delivery. Sometimes the placenta can appear to be intact and you have no excess bleeding immediately post-partum. However, if you have post-partum bleeding that lasts longer than six weeks, an investigation should be undertaken to determine if you have a fragment of retained placenta or membranes. A piece as small as ¼ inch can cause prolonged bleeding beyond six weeks post-partum.

Lacerations

Lacerations are the least common cause of post-partum hemorrhage, but when present, can be life threatening. The most common lacerations are of the perineum, vagina, and cervix.

Cervical lacerations are often the result of sudden cervical "dilation" in which the cervix tears rather than dilates. This can be due to either a "precipitous labor" or to mom pushing before full cervical dilation. Wait until your provider or nurse informs you your cervix is fully dilated before you begin to push.

Vaginal and perineal lacerations are produced by fetal malpresentation, such as a hand coming down simultaneous with the head, and from instrumented deliveries such as forceps and vacuum. Occiput posterior position of the fetal head also increases the risk of anal sphincter injury by two-to three-fold.

The cure for a laceration is to repair it. Usually this is done in the LDR. Sometimes, due to inadequate visualization or anesthesia, you will be taken to an operating room for repair of a laceration if it is a deep vaginal or cervical injury. This allows for better anesthesia and better light so your obstetric surgeon can do the best job possible for you.

Repair of lacerations stops bleeding immediately. They usually heal quickly and don't cause long-term problems. Pelvic floor dysfunctions such as unintended loss of urine and gas are the result of pressure on your pelvic muscles and nerves during pregnancy and delivery, not from lacerations.

Birth Plans Revisited

I hope I've conveyed to you that most births are normal vaginal births without complications. I also hope you understand labor and delivery is not predictable and medical interventions have been developed to maximize maternal and fetal health. Your and your baby's health is your nurses' and providers' top priority.

It is standard to allow women to walk during labor, eat in early labor, have the baby on the tummy immediately after delivery, allow dad to cut the cord, breast-feed immediately, and set whatever mood you like with music and lighting, etc. If you take prenatal classes, most include a tour of the birth place. So it is unnecessary to state these kinds of things in a birth plan.

If you are going to draw up a birth plan review it with your provider well before delivery—by thirty-six weeks gestation is ideal. Don't thrust it in their faces as you're being wheeled into the birth place in active labor.

Avoid absolutes pertaining to medical intervention such as "I don't want pitocin for delivery of the placenta." Pitocin given after the placenta comes minimizes your blood loss and risk for transfusion. This and other medical interventions have improved maternal and fetal health over the past century. These types of statements are also likely to annoy your nurses and providers because it implies you don't trust their medical judgment and it makes them feel constrained when it comes to doing the right thing for your health. They are trained professionals. Trust them.

Home Births

Some people opt for home births for a number of reasons: financial, religious, and personal. If you're planning a home birth you have the tools in this book to recognize when maternal or fetal health is in jeopardy. Monitor the fetal heart rate at least every five minutes when mom is in active labor. Develop your plan ahead of time should an emergency arise. Be cognizant of the fact that should disaster occur, by the time you get to a hospital it may be too late.

While I respect your decision to choose a home birth, I recommend for your own and your baby's safety, you deliver at a medical facility staffed by licensed nurses and obstetric providers, rather than take the route of home birth.

Water Births

Unlike fish, humans breathe air. All babies have to exit the womb eventually. The transition of the baby from a liquid to an air environment takes place within the first few seconds of life—by the fourth breath (see Science Notes in Chapter

Six). Delivery of the baby underwater does not "ease" the transition from fetus to newborn. You plan to take the baby out of the water—don't you? Reports exist in the medical literature of newborn death from drowning with underwater births.

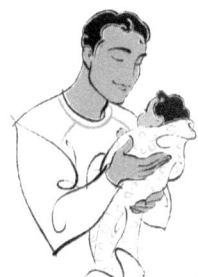

For Dads

You've been the good coach: Walking the floors of the hospital with your lady, supporting her through transition, counting for her and being her cheerleader while pushing. The baby's not coming, and you're going to C-section. All of a sudden you may feel relegated to the role of a bystander, rather than a participant. At this point you may experience a bit of a let-down—disappointment and frustration that the birth of your child has been put on hold and relocated to a foreign environment—the operating room.

Focus on the fact that this is temporary. Your most crucial role in the support of your lady and your child occurs in the weeks and months following birth, not during labor. During a C-section you're not out of the picture—you're going to be the first parent to touch your child!

You will be escorted into the operating room once your lady has a good anesthetic established. Your mere presence will allow her to feel less alone and give comfort. After the baby is born and assessed by the pediatrician, he will be bundled and given to you to present to your lady while her surgery is being completed. You and the pediatrician and baby's nurse will proceed to the nursery where your child will be measured, weighed, and you may give him his first bath.

Some maternity units will allow you to come back into the surgical recovery room to be with your lady and help her initiate breastfeeding. Welcome to fatherhood.

Office Notes: The Longest Labor

During the final week of your pregnancy you spent a lot of time daydreaming about your labor and your baby. You probably imagined a cuddly outcome with a normal delivery, the baby on your tummy, baby's father bent over your shoulder, caressing and crooning at the new life you've created. Most of you will have this birth experience and I sincerely hope you do.

Others of you may not be so lucky. You may have started contracting days before your body kicked in to true labor. Then you may have spent twenty hours in actual labor, twelve of which were active labor. You endured an hour's worth of transition. At this point you haven't slept in days. You finally get to complete cervical dilation and you're exhausted. However, you rally and push like a champ ... for ***three hours*** and the baby is not coming. (I hope at some point in this ordeal you've obtained an epidural.)

Your ob provider may or may not attempt a forceps or vacuum delivery, depending on how low the head is, chances for success, and other factors.

Ultimately you have a C-section and by the time your baby is born, you're so exhausted you have trouble mounting excitement over your child.

This birth experience feels like the worst of all worlds: a long labor, pushing forever, and still ending up in the operating room. Women who have this experience often undergo a period of grief or almost depression. They're happy with their child but they keep reliving the birth experience in an attempt to make it different. Often this grief hits without warning. It can last for days or weeks. Usually it resolves on its own as your delivery fades into the background and you focus on your infant. If you find it's not passing, talk to your ob provider.

Chapter 8

DIY, Baby! Home Birth: A New Paradigm

Disclaimer

The information presented herein is not intended to be specific medical advice or a substitute for traditional obstetric care. Consult your health care provider regarding your situation.

Home Birth—Are You Kidding—Why on Earth Would You Want to Do Home Birth?

People elect to deliver at home for many reasons. Each year in the United States, about 25,000 or 0.6 percent of all births occur in private residences. An additional 15,000 occur in free-standing "birth centers". This figure has remained stable for as long as it has been tracked, at least the past fifteen years. However, it may be time to reconsider home birth as a viable option. Early studies on home birth show it is as safe as hospital birth *for low risk women*. Those four words are essential to understand if you're considering home birth. About eighty-five percent of women can deliver safely at home (Yes, 85%!) if the proper selection criteria are used to judge whether you are a good candidate for home birth.

Unfortunately I became aware of the number of people who deliver at home through disasters. These are home deliveries gone awry over the years. I have never seen a mother or baby die over my years as an obstetrician, but I have seen women come into the hospital with bleeding from retained placentas or infection. Every woman arrived at the hospital in advance of dire emergency and no one suffered serious consequences. All the babies I've encountered through managing the aftermaths of home births have been safe, healthy, and normal.

Although I have never seen any maternal or newborn deaths from home deliveries, I cannot in good conscience recommend you undertake home birth until enough good large studies are done on it to determine it is safe. However, I can tell you through my research I've learned millions of women in developed countries deliver safely at home. Although I had previously dismissed the idea of home birth out of hand, through studying it I have come to realize it may be safer than we believed under the right circumstances.

If you're set on home birth I know you can't be talked out of it so I wish for you to do it as safely as possible.

Reasons People Desire Home Birth

Personal

Some people simply would prefer to deliver at home in their own environment, surrounded by their loved ones, without the interference of hospital personnel and other strangers.

Some people fear or dislike hospitals. They may have had a bad experience with a hospital or they associate hospitals with sickness and death. They may fear needles or doctors or nurses or have any one of several reservations about the medical environment.

Financial

Financial concerns may become a more predominant factor in the decision to deliver at home as the health care system in the United States changes. Many private insurance plans exclude maternity coverage. Many people have high deductible plans or HSA's (Health Savings Accounts) and are expected to bear a large part of maternity cost out of pocket.

Even if the nation moves to a "national" health care payer system you may decide to "opt out" for any of these reasons. Health care delivery, especially of low-risk high volume conditions such as normal labor and delivery are likely to become more "mechanized" and less personal.

Spiritual/Religious

Some people prefer to deliver at home due to religious, spiritual, or cultural concerns. For example, the Amish tend to deliver at home.

Access to Care

You may live in a rural area far from a hospital or birth center. Or your access to medical care may be limited by finances. In the near future maternity care is likely to become more centralized. More obstetricians are quitting the business due to lifestyle and malpractice issues, as well as declining reimbursement.

Within the next decade it is foreseeable labor and delivery services may be provided by a "hospitalist"—a certified nurse midwife or physician who only works in the hospital in shifts. You'd see a "regular" doctor or midwife for your prenatal care and then be delivered by the "obstetric hospitalist" on call. You likely won't know who is delivering your baby prior to labor. You may not even meet them until you're in labor. You're likely to have more than one "hospitalist" attend your birth due to change of shifts.

Home Birth: Safer Than You Think

A truly astounding phenomenon has occurred in the United States over the past hundred years. I'll name that phenomenon the "medicalization of the extremes of life: birth and death". Somehow we've come to believe as a culture that one must be born and die in a hospital. Or, if not actually in the hospital, with a hospital somehow involved in close proximity. Family members congregate at the hospital to witness and participate in the drama of hospital-based birth and death. When and why did we allow the hospital to become the setting for the most sacred life rituals, birth and death?

The gold standard in medical science research is the "randomized double blinded controlled trial" (RDBCT's). This is a type of study in which a drug, procedures, or treatment is compared to placebo (or non-intervention) by blinding a "control" group and a "study" group to the type of treatment, and comparing outcomes. Any modern treatment must undergo the rigors of the RBDCT's in order to be accepted in the armamentarium of allopathic medical treatment.

Never has a randomized controlled study been done on whether it is safer or preferable to be born and/or die at home versus in a hospital. On the other hand, hundreds of observational studies have shown that ninety percent of the health care dollar is spent in the final six months of life and a large portion of the remaining ten percent is spent on "million dollar" premature babies.

Contrary to conventional wisdom hospitals may not be the ideal place in which to be born or die. In fact prior to the discovery of the "germ theory of disease" maternal mortality was much higher for mother who delivered in the hospital due to transmission of a lethal bacteria, Group A Streptococcus, from one laboring mother to another by medical personnel who failed to wash their hands or use gloves between examining patients. Ignaz Semmelweiz is credited for identifying this factor in the early nineteenth century as a significant cause of maternal mortality. As with many geniuses, when he made his initial postulation he was laughed out of the medical community and ostracized as a "nut case". Eventually hospital staff and colleagues "came around" to understand his point of view and the use of "aseptic technique" (hand washing, sterile gloves, sterile prep for surgery and other measures) were adopted as the "standard of care".

Many other procedures have been incorporated into the standard of care in obstetrics without proof that these measures reduce fetal, neonatal, or maternal morbidity and mortality. For example, nearly every woman laboring in a U.S. hospital gets an intravenous, continuous external fetal monitoring, and "put to bed" to labor. Although the latter is declining—many hospitals now allow women to walk and use a hot tub during labor—the former two practices are in full force and showing no evidence of declining or being used in a rational way. Because of their acceptance as "standard of care" many obstetric practitioners and hospitals refuse to deviate from these practices due to fear of lawsuits. Thus, current obstetric practice is driven by forces that have no basis in rational scientific study.

Although it is becoming less common, laboring women must subvert their own wisdom, knowledge, and intuition to "professionally trained" doctors, midwives, and nurses. Having been trained in and practiced in the American medical system since 1992 I began to question the validity of the present model several years ago for many reasons, the foremost of which was a desire to honor my patients' wisdom and wishes regarding the birth of her child. I question many of the practices we hold as "sacred" in modern obstetrics and I wonder if there is a better, more dignified, less expensive, way to give birth in the United States.

Indeed, a study reported in the New England Journal of Medicine several years ago revealed that continuous external fetal monitoring actually increases the cesarean delivery compared to fetuses who are monitored "intermittently" or every five minutes during the hardest phase of labor. Although this study was well done, its results have not been incorporated into clinical medicine due to fear of lawsuits on the part of clinicians.

Prior to modern medicine the maternal and fetal mortality rate was roughly twenty-five percent. However, this mortality rate was due to many factors that modern studies of home birth have shown can be safely identified and managed at home, or transferred to hospital care if necessary: hemorrhage, obstructed labor, pregnancy-induced high blood pressure, fetal intolerance to labor, and fetal "malpresentation" such as breech (butt first).

Since the 1980's several other "first world" countries have initiated the practice of home birth with trained certified nurse midwives as birth attendants. This practice is most widespread in Canada but also exists in the Netherlands, Great Britain, and Australia to name others. In third world countries such as Africa and Afghanistan, most births are conducted at home and the struggle in these regions is to get trained personnel out to rural areas to help women identify and deal with complications of labor and delivery.

The largest study of maternal and neonatal outcomes for women who choose home birth was conducted in Canada and reported in the British Medical Journal in 2005. This study looked at 5,418 women who elected to have a home birth in the year 2000 with a midwife certified by the North American Registry of Midwives as a birth attendant. These birth attendants undergo similar training involving an apprenticeship as do Certified Nurse Midwives in the United States. However, for the option of home birth there are protocols identified and followed for maternal and fetal transport to hospital care should a complication arise.

The study compared the 5400 women who elected home birth with the 3.3 million hospital births that occurred in the United States during the year 2000. The results of the Canadian study are eye-opening: Of the five thousand women, *eighty-eight percent* of them delivered successfully at home with a health mom and baby.

Twelve percent of the women were transported to the hospital for the following reasons: over half for failure to progress in labor (failure of the cervix to dilate and the baby to descend into the pelvis), pain relief, or maternal exhaustion—all non-emergent conditions. Life threatening emergencies such as fetal intolerance of labor, prolapse of the umbilical cord, and maternal hemorrhage, accounted for less than two percent of transfers combined. Other reasons for transfer included newborn respiratory problems, breech position, and retained placenta.

The intrapartum mortality rate (death rate of the fetus during labor) for home births was 1.7/1000, *identical to that of the 3.3 million in-hospital term births in the United States.*

Once transported to the hospital the following medical interventions were undertaken in the home-birth group versus the hospital-labored group: continuous electronic fetal monitoring (9.6% compared to 84.3% in the hospital-labored group); episiotomy (2.1% versus 33% in the hospital-labored group), cesarean section (3.7% versus 19% in the hospital-labored group), vacuum extraction (0.6% versus 5.5% in the hospital-labored group). The cesarean section rate among women attempting home birth was 8.3% among women who were having their first birth and 1.6% among women who had delivered prior infants. For reference, the present (2006) cesarean section rate in the United States is 30.6%.

Moreover, Canadian women attempting home birth reported a much greater satisfaction with their birth experience, even if they were among the twelve percent who were transported for hospital intervention. They described their home birth experience with a trained attendant as more "relaxing", less "stressful" and allowing a greater role for the father of the baby or their significant other.

The Canadian study is the largest and most recent look at home birth attended by a trained professional. Several studies from Canada, Great Britain, Australia, the Netherlands, and other countries exist dating back to the 1980's. Some of these studies, particularly those of Australian home births found an increase in maternal and neonatal mortality but these were attributed to delayed recognition of emergent conditions by the birth attendant. The Australian birth attendants in those studies had not undergone the same rigorous training as had the Canadian birth attendants in 2000.

The Canadian study is the largest study on home birth to date. Some studies have shown home birth is "as safe" as hospital birth; while other studies (e.g. Australian study) have shown home birthed babies have higher mortality rates. Although these studies have conflicting results, it is likely due to the

> **Home birth may be safe if the following conditions are met:**
> - The pregnancy is "low risk".
> - The birth attendant is skilled in managing labor and complications of labor.
> - The birth occurs in close proximity to a hospital.
> - The mother has had a previous successful vaginal birth.

different sizes of the studies and the different levels of training of the home birth attendants in the studies. However, despite these apparent discrepancies some clear conclusions can be drawn about home birth:

Home birth is a safe option for low risk women if they are attended by a skilled birth attendant and done close enough to a hospital to deal with an emergency should one arise.

The findings of the Canadian study fly in the face of everything "indoctrinated" into American birth attendants and American women in general. In the current climate of medical finances and medical malpractice the possibility is remote that home birth with trained attendants will be given serious study in the next decade.

However, I believe all these issues, plus the findings of the Canadian study show home birth deserves further evaluation in the United States. Perhaps there is a better, less expensive, more loving way to bring a child into the world; just as there may be less costly, more dignified way to exit this world and pass into the one beyond …

How do we get from where we are now in the highly technical to a rational approach to home birth or at least minimalist intervention hospital birth? In a stepwise fashion that looks at pregnancy and birth within a wellness mind frame, and not as a "medical condition" or state of illness that must be endured or overcome.

The ideal candidate for home birth:
- **Has no underlying medical illnesses such as diabetes or high blood pressure**
- **Can get to a hospital in less than twenty minutes**
- **Has had previous normal births**
- **Is of normal weight and has a normal size baby**
- **Has support people**
- **Is attended by a person trained in management of labor and its complications**
- **Won't panic in an emergency**
- **Is willing to abandon the attempt early on if baby or mom is in jeopardy**
- **Can recognize if baby or mom is in jeopardy**

Are you a good physical candidate to attempt home birth?

The ideal candidate for a home birth would be a woman of normal weight who's had one or two successful vaginal births under her belt. She would know what to expect from labor as far as her pain tolerance, duration of labor, and she'd have confidence in her ability to deliver vaginally. Each successive labor becomes shorter than the one before it, unless there is a major difference between pregnancies. For example if Marcy gained 30 lbs with her first birth and had a 7 lb girl, but with her second pregnancy she gained 60 lbs, she's more likely to have a large baby (passenger) and a more difficult labor.

If you're considering home birth it's essential you assess your physical condition realistically—you're neither under or overweight; you've had good nutrition throughout pregnancy; and you have maintained your muscle strength and endurance with moderate exercise throughout pregnancy.

It is also a good idea to have your partner or birth attendant assess your clinical pelvimetry (as described in Chapter Six) to determine if your pelvis is roomy enough to deliver vaginally or if it is not.

If you're going to attempt home birth preparation is essential. You must be willing to assemble supplies and locate a birth attendant. You must also have a tolerance for mess. The average blood loss with a normal vaginal birth is about one-half to one liter. There's also the placenta to contend with. Identify a clean, well-lit place to deliver. Assemble towels and clothes you can use for labor that can be discarded later if they become soiled.

Green Light: Home Birth Attempt is a "Go" if You …
- Identify you're a good candidate (low risk) and have consulted a licensed health care provider to confirm this.
- Are motivated and have a strong desire to deliver at home.
- Have a skilled birth attendant—preferably a certified nurse midwife or physician if you can get one to attend your birth.
- Have proximity to a hospital (less than twenty minutes).
- Have an emergency plan of which all support people are aware and have "rehearsed".
- Have an ability to recognize a deteriorating situation before it becomes a dire emergency.
- Are willing to abandon the home birth attempt should you or your baby's health be in jeopardy.

Are You a Good Mental/Emotional Candidate for Home Birth?

Not only are you motivated; you are realistic. You are prepared. You've assembled the necessary supplies and people and you've formulated one or two emergency plans for "what if" scenarios. Take into account the time of year you'll be delivering and acknowledge any challenges the weather may present.

If an emergency arises you won't panic—you'll engage your abdominal breathing and execute the steps of your emergency plan you and your birth attendants have rehearsed.

You're not "married" to your home birth plan. If it's not working, you're willing to abandon your plan, even if it means disappointment. You won't feel guilty or like a failure if it doesn't work out. You can have a "take it as it comes" attitude.

Establish Relationships Prior to Delivery

If possible, identify a professional licensed health care provider for you and your baby. Most licensed physicians and certified nurse midwives will not agree to be available for your home delivery for the simple reason they don't want to incur the liability. However, if possible you should at least have a relationship with someone possessing obstetric expertise and someone able to care for a newborn should the need arise.

Contraindications to Attempting Home Birth

If you are "high risk" (see box) you are NOT a good candidate for attempting home birth. Locate a competent physician or certified nurse midwife in whom you have utmost confidence and enjoy being a healthy mom and having a healthy baby. You can change your risk status by maintaining a normal weight, exercising before, during and after pregnancy; and observing a healthy lifestyle incorporating a stress management program.

Who should attend your birth?

Ideally a licensed medical professional such as a certified nurse midwife or physician should attend your home birth. At present you are unlikely to find this, although that doesn't preclude this service being available in the future.

There are many "lay midwives" and doulas available. These are people who lack formal medical training but have an interest in birth. They have sometimes studied abroad or in the United States to gain expertise in management of labor and delivery. Some are actually quite experienced and qualified, while others are simply dangerous out of lack of knowledge and expertise. Interview your prospective lay midwife or doula. How many births have they done? What is their training? What percent of their patients are transferred to hospital care and for what reasons?

At the minimum, your birth attendant should:

➢ Be able to transport you to the hospital if needed

➢ Be able to keep a level head in an emergency

➢ Be supportive of your choices should you wish to abandon the home birth attempt due to medical reasons or a lack of pain control or any other circumstance that should arise.

➢ Not be squeamish; can tolerated mess and the sight of blood without passing out.

If you can't find a birth attendant(s) who meet these criteria, you should deliver at a hospital.

RED LIGHT: **Home birth is a "NO GO" if you have:**
- **Multiple fetuses (twins)**
- **Heart Disease**
- **Kidney Disease**
- **Pre-eclampsia or Pregnancy-Induced Hypertension**
- **Diabetes (insulin-dependent or gestational)**
- **Breech or other abnormal position of fetus**
- **Bleeding after 20 weeks gestation**
- **Previous C-section**
- **Age under fifteen or over forty**
- **No support system (at least one trained labor attendant and one other support person)**
- **Are unwilling to abandon the attempted home birth should complications arise**
- **Have no transportation to hospital**
- **Live > 20 minutes from hospital**

Preparation is Key: Supplies Necessary for Home Birth

Before you decide whether or not to attempt home birth ask yourself if you can gather the necessary supplies and make sure you understand the concept of "sterile technique".

Semmelweis made the famous discovery that "childbed fever," a deadly womb infection, is caused by bacteria called "Group A Strep". Childbed fever was transmitted in hospitals by doctors and nurses who examined successive patients without washing their hands in-between. If you plan to deliver at home it is crucial you use sterile gloves, instruments, and towels for touching mom or baby. You must possess the capacity to sterilize these things, or be able to order pre-sterilized from a medical supply distributor.

Birth supplies:
- **Common sense**
- **Fetal Doppler**
- **Sterile gloves**
- **Sterile towels**
- **Sterile clamps, scissors, and suture**
- **Bulb suction device**
- **Cytotec (misoprostol) if you can get it**
- **Common sense**

Part of controlling infection is to minimize the number of cervical exams done. You should examine mom's cervix no more than every two hours. If mom has entered active labor and there is no cervical change over a two hour period it is time to go to the hospital for failure to progress in labor. You don't necessarily need a cesarean section, but at the hospital the staff can administer you medication to increase the strength of your contractions, and possible enable you to finish out your labor normally. The risk of infection is directly proportional to the number of cervical exams: the more cervical exams done, the higher the risk of infection.

Other sterile supplies necessary are gloves, towels, cord clamps, scissors, suture, a suture needle driver, and hemostats.

Essential to any birth is a Doppler fetal heart rate monitor. These can now be purchased in many department stores, through the Internet, and pregnancy magazines. You must check the fetal heart rate every fifteen minutes in early labor and every five minutes in hard labor and during pushing. If at any time the fetal heart rate drops below 120 beats per minute for more than one minute you should proceed to the hospital. Likewise, if the fetal heart rate stays above 160 beats per minute for thirty minutes or more, you should proceed to the hospital.

Labor at Home:
- **Use common sense**
- **Anticipate**
- **Don't panic**
- **Study chapters Six and Seven**

In the advent of post-partum hemorrhage, if you can obtain misoprostol (Cytotec) prior to labor, administer 800 micrograms (eight tablets) via the rectum. Misoprostol is a prostaglandin or chemical that aids in contraction of the uterus. It has very few side effects and can resolve a life-threatening situation.

Managing Labor at Home

Be vigilant and proactive. Learn to recognize a deteriorating situation before it devolves into an emergency. Be willing

Common sense is crucial.

to go to the hospital. If you're uncertain whether or not you should go—just go!

For mom's comfort use all the positions shown in chapter seven for pain management and to "get through" the average twelve hours of labor.

The fetal heart rate normally fluctuates in labor. It increases with fetal movement and can decrease with fetal rest periods or with brief compression of the umbilical cord. The fetal heart rate also changes with maternal position. If you notice a drop in the fetal heart rate, try lying on your left side, getting on your hands and knees, or walking while you are evaluating whether the heart rate is staying low long enough to proceed to the hospital. Be proactive—don't wait for the baby to have a sustained drop in heart rate (fewer than 120 beats per minute for longer than one minute) to make preparations to proceed to the hospital.

The only exception to this rule is if the baby is literally about to come out and has a drop in heart rate. Sometimes just as the baby's head is "crowning" and about to deliver, the heart rate will drop. In this case it may be necessary to stimulate the baby after birth by massaging her feet and back.

Take deep breaths. Avoid hyperventilation. If you find your hands and feet tingling or you're getting dizzy, short of breath, or light headed, these are symptoms of hyperventilation. Slow your breathing down and try to breathe from your abdomen and not high in your chest.

Study chapters seven and eight to learn the steps of normal labor and to recognize when things aren't proceeding normally.

Once the baby is delivered there is no hurry to clamp and cut the cord as long as mom is not bleeding heavily and the baby is breathing well. On the other hand do not forget, in the excitement, to clamp and cut the cord. I normally put the baby on mom's abdomen and wait until the cord stops "pulsing" to clamp and cut it. There is no "right" way to clamp and cut the cord, other than to make sure both ends are securely clamped prior to doing it so as to avoid unnecessary blood loss from mom or babe.

Delivery of the Placenta

The placenta normally delivers spontaneously about twenty minutes after the baby. It can take up to forty-five minutes, but anything greater than one hour is definitely abnormal. Go to the hospital if the placenta is not delivering.

Do not pull on the umbilical cord! You will cause the cord to break, and the placenta will remain stuck in mom's womb. If necessary, you can reach into the vagina (with sterile gloved hands), and if you can feel the placenta bulging through the cervix, you can grasp the leading edge of the placenta and gently pull it out. This is normally not necessary and if you're thinking of doing this, plan how you'll get to the hospital should it not work.

Massage the uterus from the outside of mom's abdomen after the placenta is out. This is called "fundal massage" and it encourages the uterus muscle to contract around the blood vessels to stop bleeding. If the uterus "relaxes" and you notice increased bleeding, do fundal massage until the uterus is firm again.

Dealing with Heavy Bleeding

Normal blood loss for a vaginal birth is about a quart. If mom is losing more than this or has sustained (lasting more than three minutes) brisk, heavy bleeding, she needs to go to the hospital. While you're making preparations to go to the hospital, look for sources of bleeding and try to mitigate them on the way.

If fundal massage isn't working, the uterus is firm, and there is still bleeding, look for a laceration (tear) of the vagina or cervix. If you feel comfortable with it you can try to throw a few sutures to close the tear long enough to stop the bleeding and have it properly repaired at the hospital. Other measures to stop bleeding are: applying pressure, "packing" the vagina and uterus with gauze or sterile towels, and applying a hemostat if you can identify a specific bleeding vessel or tear. If you are employing these measures, make sure you're also going to the hospital to have things properly evaluated and treated.

> **Sources and treatment of bleeding at home:**
> - **"Boggy" uterus—fundal massage; if you have it on hand, administer misoprostol 800 mcg via the rectum**
> - **Tear of vagina or cervix—apply pressure, clamp, pack or suture the tear**

If you can obtain misoprostol (Cytotec) prior to labor, administer 800 micrograms (eight tablets) via the rectum. Misoprostol is a prostaglandin or chemical that aids in contraction of the uterus. It has very few side effects and can resolve a life-threatening situation. (This is repeated here because it is important!)

Keep Your Eye on the Ball

Remember the goals are a healthy mom and baby. No one wins an award for her mode or place of delivery. Keep a level head and have a safe and healthy pregnancy, birth, mom, and baby.

Chapter 9

A Perfect Love, A Perfect Life: Newborn and Post-partum Period

A Love Like No Other

You've done it! You're holding your new baby in your arms and she's perfect. Maybe she looks more like you or her dad, or an equal combination of both; regardless, she's beautiful. You're flooded with love like none you've ever experienced. You can't imagine caring for another person with this depth or intensity. You *get it*—"unconditional love". You want to nurture and protect this person, help them grow into a full-fledged human being. You wish you could will away global problems—war, famine, climate change. You want the planet to be a perfect place so your child will never face any danger or threat. You desire nothing less than world peace.

The First Week Post Partum

Other than recovering from birth, the first forty eight hours may seem like a piece of cake. Most babies sleep nearly continuously for the first two days. *You're* exhausted from labor and delivery—well so are *they*. When awake, most newborns just look around and take it all in. Babies gradually become more interactive by six weeks of age.

Usually you have to physically stimulate newborns to wake up and eat the first two days. When you finally get them latched on, they often fall asleep. Normal newborns lose ten percent of their body weight by one week of age. Don't worry—they gain it back, and then some by six weeks. For specific details on breast-feeding refer to that section in this chapter.

By two or three days most of you are home from the hospital—thank goodness. You've had it with hospital meals and nurses mashing on your abdomen to "check your fundus". After the first forty eight hours your baby will gradually establish a routine of eating, sleeping, and pooping. Most babies sleep longer during the day and wake more frequently at night. This pattern is tough on parents, but it's normal for newborns. Usually by six weeks of age babies have switched their days and nights to sleep more consistently at night. Once your baby's routine is established, your life is more predictable.

However, "predictable" does not equal "easy". "What were we thinking?" You may wonder at times during this week. Remember this: *Sleep when you can*. Sleep deprivation magnifies any negative emotions you're experiencing. It also decreases your coping skills.

You may be inundated with relatives and well-wishers. Dealing with company is stressful when you have a new baby and you're exhausted. If you're overwhelmed by visitors, explain you're tired, thank them for coming and invite them to come by in a few weeks. Inform them that they can really be of help by dropping off a meal—food that reheats easily like lasagna or casseroles.

You're finally settled at home. You've learned your baby's patterns and can anticipate his needs. You've figured out to sleep when the baby sleeps. This isn't so bad—is it? Then all hell breaks loose. Just when you're gaining confidence as a parent *it* strikes: The first night of *inconsolable crying*.

It usually happens at one or two weeks of age. Some parents are blessed with just a few of these; others struggle with them night after night for the first three months. Either way, it shakes your confidence and makes you wonder if you (and your new baby) will live to see it through.

Inconsolable Crying (Colic)

This phenomenon of inconsolable crying is often still referred to as *colic*. Nobody knows what "colic" really is. "Colic" is often attributed to painful intestinal gas as the baby's digestive sys-

> **Most "colic" resolves by three month of age.**

tem is maturing. However, medication to dissolve gas bubbles such as simethicone (Mylicon) drops, do not produce a miracle cure for colic, and may have no effect whatsoever. Furthermore, there's no medical science to support intestinal gas as the sole cause for "colic".

In desperation you'll explore every avenue imaginable to appease your inconsolable baby. Whatever you do—*do not* allow your baby use your breast as a 24-7 pacifier. You'll wind up with excruciatingly painful nipples, sleep deprivation, and possibly resentment and depression. Seek out other techniques.

Some babies respond to a specific hold or position, such as draped over your lap on their tummies (no—not both your hands around their neck). A car ride or a session on top of the clothes dryer in their car seat may be the magic cure for some. Most babies are calmed by skin-to-skin contact. Some babies don't seem to have "solutions" and just have to cry it out until they exhaust themselves. Be advised: There's no sound in the natural world more unsettling and stress-inducing than that of a baby crying out of control.

If none of the "tricks" work, there are generally two philosophies on dealing with babies who can't be consoled at night: The "let them cry it out" approach; and the "family bed" approach. Often babies just need the comfort of your skin and body heat—remember they spent their first nine months inside your warm cozy body—the outside world can be a harsh transition. Depending on his or her philosophy, your pediatrician may advise you to leave the baby in her crib and let her "cry it out". This failed for us.

Our first baby was "colicky"–night after night of inconsolable crying. This usually began at 7:00 PM and lasted until 3:00 AM or longer. We tried all the tricks. My husband walked him around the apartment or spent hours at 2:00 AM driving around a crying boy to get him to sleep only to have him waken when he was brought into the apartment. His only consistent soother seemed to be nursing and skin-to-skin contact. After lots of blind alleys, exhausted to the brink of insanity, we caved and unofficially adopted the "family bed" approach. Be forewarned some studies have suggested the "family bed" approach is associated with a higher rate of SIDS (sudden infant death syndrome). This link remains controversial.

It was a war of attrition—no one got any sleep with the baby screaming, and the only measure that seemed to calm him was skin-to-skin contact. When he reached an age where he could physically get out of bed, he did so, and climbed into our bed every night. He didn't stop sleeping in our bed until he was four, when our daughter was born. (You may ask why did we ever have a second one? Parental brain damage.) Our daughter was much easier on us and quit sleeping in our bed when she was weaned at ten months of age. We didn't realize how chronically tired we were those first five years until after our daughter quit sleeping in our bed and we got more consistent sleep.

Your ultimate goal is to have a secure, well-adjusted child. Whatever it takes to get there is the "right" thing to do. You'll know from your baby's response whether he will be able to "cry it out" or if you're going to have to resort to other measures such as the family bed.

Pacifiers and Artificial Nipples

Save yourself some grief and introduce your baby to a pacifier. Pacifiers come in many sizes and shapes; some bear the official approval of the American Dental Association. No randomized controlled double-blinded study has shown which pacifier is universally best. Your baby will usually develop a preference for a specific pacifier. Purchase at least ten of these and store them in strategic places where they'll always be handy—the car, the crib, the kitchen, by the phone, the diaper changing center, etc.

Training your baby to accept an artificial nipple will also allow dad and others to help out more with feeding the baby pumped breast milk or formula. This will allow mom to have a break and perhaps get out of the house for a walk or some other personal time. Build time into your schedule for self rejuvenation. A new baby takes it all out of you. Find a way to replenish yourself—whether it's through exercise, a long bath, meditation, browsing the mall, whatever.

Babies tend to be accepting of pacifiers and artificial nipples if they are initiated before four weeks of age. Your baby usually won't develop a "nipple preference" as long as you introduce a pacifier or artificial nipple early. However, by one month of age many babies have established specific neuromuscular patterns for suckling because they're used to whatever they've been given in the first four weeks. Offer your baby several nipples of differing shapes and sizes—the real thing for breast-feeding, a pacifier for comfort suckling, and an artificial nipple to allow another person to feed the baby pumped milk or formula. Teaching your baby to be adaptable by four weeks of age will serve her well for her entire life.

Breast-feeding and Lactation

Step One: Latch-On

Rewind back to the first moments of your child's life. By ten to twenty minutes the newborn usually calms down and begins to "root" or rhythmically move her tongue about in search of a

> **A wide open mouth is essential to successful infant latch-on.**

nipple. It's time to try latching on. With proper latch-on technique, the baby applies her lips to the areola with a wide open mouth and your nipple presses against her palate. This stimulates coordinated suckling motion of the tongue. After a minute or two of suckling you may feel your milk "let-down".

The key to successful latch-on is to get the baby to open her mouth as wide as possible so she grips the areola with her mouth, and not the actual nipple. With the lips contacting the areola, the actual nipple is inserted well in the baby's mouth against the palate. The pressure of the nipple on the palate stimulates babies to engage in proper suckling. A wide open mouth applied to the areola is essential to successful breastfeeding.

Newborns need to *learn* how to latch on—they're not very coordinated at first. They have the instincts but haven't established the muscle control. Sometimes the best way to get her to learn latch on correctly is to wait until she's mid-wail and "pop" her on or stuff the nipple into her wide open mouth. She'll automatically begin suckling, and eventually she'll learn to open her mouth wide to latch on.

Try not to let her "chew" her way on, as that will result in cracked and painful nipples. If she's not latching on with a wide open mouth, detach her by sliding your finger between her lips and your nipple and try again. Repeat the process until she gets it right. You'll know because the pressure of her mouth will be on your areola, not on the tip of your nipple.

Another crucial element to proper latch-on is a supple areola. If your breasts are engorged, the areola becomes taut and won't conform to the baby's mouth during latch on—imagine trying to hold a fully inflated balloon in your mouth. If engorged, pump your breast a little to empty it before trying to latch on until the areola is flexible enough to conform to the baby's mouth as he latches on.

Inverted and Flat Nipples

With good latch-on and suckling technique, a baby will naturally draw out an inverted or flat nipple. Once he's gripped the areola, his suckling action will pull the nipple into his mouth. Most women with inverted or flat nipples can successfully breast-feed.

If you're having trouble establishing latch-on due to inverted nipples you can use a breast pump to draw out the nipple, then initiate latch on. See more about inverted nipples under "Nipple Problems".

What is breast milk and when does it "come in"?

For two to three days after delivery you produce colostrum. Colostrum is a watery mixture of sugars, proteins, and immunity molecules. It's perfect for your baby's immature digestive system. Colostrum is not produced in large volumes—your baby may only consume three ounces per day.

Between three to five days after birth your milk "comes in". You may experience engorgement or sudden swelling of the breasts as the milk comes in. When your milk comes in you may suddenly start leaking profusely. Some women get a fever as their milk comes in. As long as it's not associated with an area of breast redness or pain, this fever is not mastitis. The breast skin may take on a bluish tinge due to dilation of the veins underneath the skin.

While breast milk contains many of the components of colostrum, it contains more fat and proteins and less sugar than colostrum. The fat in breast milk promotes your baby's brain and nerve development.

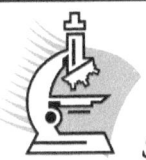

Science Notes: Composition of Breast Milk; Why "Breast is Best"

Breast milk is the perfect food for your infant from birth through six months. After six months solids need to be introduced to complement the nutrition in breast milk. Most commercial formulas are based on cow's milk or soy milk. Formula is adequate but breast milk is superb. Here's why:

Fats: Human breast milk contains more of the essential fatty acids necessary for brain and nerve development, than does cow's milk. These fatty acids include oleic acid, palmitic acid; linoleic, linolenic acids; arachidonic and docosahexanoic acids. These are "long-chain fatty acids" essential to development of human brain and nerve cells. In comparison, cow's milk contains fewer of these essential fatty acids, in lower amounts. Cow's milk contains a higher proportion of "short chain fatty acids".

Proteins: Human colostrum contains a high proportion of Immunoglobulin A (IgA) which coats the baby's digestive system and provides protection from diseases to which the mother has developed immunity. Cow's milk contains predominantly IgG which is broken down by the human digestive system and does not provide as much immune protection. The main proteins in human milk are casein and whey in a ratio of 60:40. The main proteins in cow's milk are casein and whey in a ration of 80:20. The increased casein in cow's milk binds calcium and creates a larger "curd" in the human baby's stomach. This decreases the availability of other micronutrients in formula versus breast milk.

Sugars: Human breast milk contains double the lactose versus cow's milk. Lactose is a complex sugar composed of glucose and galactose. Cow's milk contains a higher proportion of smaller sugar molecules.

Other Components of Human Milk: Human breast milk contains growth modulators; white blood cells to fight infection; digestive enzymes; cytokines, a different type of immune molecule than immunoglobulins; and different proportions of micronutrients such as calcium, zinc, chloride, phosphorus, and potassium than cow's milk.

Human Milk Changes Over Time: Colostrum, produced for the first three days, is mostly water, protein (Immunoglobulin A and Lactoferrin – two immune proteins), and some sugars. Colostrum is produced in a low volume of about three ounces per day. It also has laxative properties to allow your baby to pass meconium ("stool" made *in utero*) and excrete excess bilirubin, the chemical that causes neonatal jaundice.

Transitional Milk, produced from about day three to ten after birth, contains gradually more fats and sugars and less proteins.

Mature Milk, produced after day ten, contains proteins, sugars, and fats. The "foremilk" or first milk is largely proteins and sugars, while the "hindmilk", produced at the end of a feeding, contains proportionally more fatty acids and proteins.

For more detailed information on composition of breast milk, visit the Centers for Disease Control website, www.cdc.gov; and the United Nations educational website, www.unu.edu and search "breast milk" or http://www.unu.edu/unupress/food/8F174e/8F174E00.htm#Contents.

Final benefits of breastfeeding: It's cheaper and less hassle than purchasing and mixing formula. It comes prepackaged at the perfect temperature, and you can't beat the presentation. Bon Appétit!

Milk Let-Down

Milk let down is the opening of ducts within the breast to allow the milk to flow to and through the nipple. It causes a tingling or pulling sensation and is due to the contraction of thousands of little muscles surrounding the milk glands and ducts. As these muscles contract, they also exert pull on the ligamentous support of the breast. During the first few weeks of lactation, you'll also get uterine cramps and increased vaginal bleeding as the milk is letting down. This is because the same hormone that triggers milk let-down, oxytocin also stimulates your uterus to contract. It's beneficial because it allows your uterus to rid itself of clots and debris.

Milk let down is stimulated by a signal from your brain—an oxytocin surge as the baby begins to latch on. It can also be triggered by manipulation of the breasts (i.e. with sex) and a shower. It can even be set off by thinking about the baby while you're at work, or engaged in some other activity. You'll probably want to purchase milk pads to place between your bra and nipple so as to prevent unscheduled (not related to a feeding) milk let-down from soaking your shirt.

Foremilk and Hindmilk: Empty One Breast Fully Before Switching

During a nursing session the milk actually changes composition. The first milk that comes out, foremilk, is watery, sugary and has some proteins in it. After about five minutes of nursing the hind-

> Foremilk contains proteins and sugars; hindmilk contains more fats.

milk is released. Hindmilk is rich with healthy fats and proteins. The hindmilk is the cream—the good stuff that will make your baby grow and put on the pounds.

Hindmilk is brain food. In addition to other things, your baby needs those fats as building blocks to make the myelin sheaths for nerves, coatings analogous to insulation on wires. As the nerves become more myelinated, the baby's muscle coordination improves. Increased myelination is responsible for babies gaining head control by six weeks and can eventually sitting up by age six months.

You should allow the baby to fully empty one breast at each feeding. This takes about fifteen minutes. Full emptying stimulates the breast to produce more complete milk—foremilk and hindmilk—for the next feeding. If you switch off before the hindmilk is emptied, eventually the breast will produce less hindmilk.

If the baby still seems hungry after emptying one side, go ahead and switch him to the other. If not, start with the side not nursed at the most recent feeding.

Asymmetry in Production and Size

Most people find that one breast produces more milk than the other—sometimes as much as twice as much. This is due to an intrinsic difference in breast size and gland number that is not so noticeable when you're not pregnant. It can also be accentuated by the baby developing a preference for one side over the other. This may be because the baby finds one side easier to latch onto, or you unconsciously hold the baby in a more comfortable position on one side versus the other.

I suggest waiting to purchase a nursing bra until your milk comes in. Your breast size can change dramatically and a bra you bought the last trimester of pregnancy can be too small. A nursing bra that is too small will make you miserable. Get a bra that comfortably fits the largest breast.

Setting

It's crucial to successful breast-feeding that you have a comfortable place to nurse. Sit in a chair or rocker that's not too tall for you. Prop your feet on a short stool to avoid overarching your spine. Having your knees slightly elevated also enables you to gently curl over the baby to make the breast more accessible.

Nursing places a lot of strain on the neck, upper back, and shoulders. Use regular pillows or a crescent shaped nursing pillow to support the baby's weight so you're not lifting the baby or bearing his weight as he's feeding. If you experience neck or shoulder pain after nursing, evaluate your body support system and make adjustments.

Nursing accessories such as pillows, rockers, stools, nipple shields, and breast pumps can be found at maternity stores, many "big box" stores, or online at the Medela website.

If you need to nurse in public maintain your privacy by throwing a shawl or blanket over you and the baby.

Nursing Holds

The two most common holds are the "cradle" hold with baby lying on his side against your thighs (supported by a pillow); and the "football" hold with the baby lying on his back, tucked under one of your arms with his neck supported by your hand while he's suckling. Within two weeks you'll develop a feel for which hold works best for you. You may even use both with equal frequency, or the cradle hold for one side and the football hold for the other side as you experiment and get more comfortable with the options.

Some important things about the nursing hold are: 1) the baby's neck is in a neutral position, and the chin not turned to face one shoulder; 2) you're not experiencing neck or back strain with the hold; 3) the baby's weight is supported by the furniture or pillows rather than you "lifting" the baby to the breast.

Frequency of Nursing: How to Tell if Your Baby's Getting Enough

Once they're past the forty-eight hour mark babies will nurse every two to three hours. This gradually extends to every three to four hours by twelve weeks of age. As long as your baby is making eight to ten wet diapers per day and gaining weight after the first week of life, he's getting enough milk. If you have concerns about your milk supply consult your pediatrician and/or certified lactation specialist.

Duration of Nursing Sessions: Nourishment vs. Comfort Nursing

Usually by a week of age the baby can empty a breast in ten to fifteen minutes. Many babies like to do "comfort" nursing where they use your nipple as a pacifier. They may

> **Succumbing to "comfort nursing" may eventually exhaust you.**

want to lounge on the breast for forty-five minutes to an hour. If you succumb to comfort nursing at every feeding you will never be free—you will be constantly engaged, develop very sore nipples leading to exhaustion, frustration, and possibly resentment and discontinuation of breastfeeding.

Do yourself a favor and use a pacifier. As long as pacifiers are introduced before a baby reaches a month of age, he generally does not develop "nipple confusion" or a "nipple preference". The same applies to nipples for bottles.

Milk Supply; Breast Pumps

Milk supply has a daily rhythm. It is greatest in the morning and tapers off by late afternoon/evening. This is due to cyclic fluctuations in the milk-producing hormone, prolactin. Prolactin is made by the brain and stimulates milk production. It is highest in the wee hours of the morning, and lowest in the afternoon/evening.

Initially your breasts may produce more milk than the baby needs. Sometimes they don't produce enough. You can use a breast pump to address either issue. A double electric breast pump is essential if you need to increase your supply or plan on returning to work before wean-

> **A double electric pump is most efficient and effective at emptying the breasts.**

ing the baby. Hand pumps only empty one breast at a time and they usually retrieve less milk from the breast than the suction exerted by an electric pump. With a double electric pump you can empty both breasts within fifteen minutes, a necessity if you're pumping on a work break. The best double electric pump I've found is the Medela Pump-N-Style. I used one myself for two babies and have given many as baby shower gifts. It's efficient and compact.

Assess your supply by the number of diapers per day your baby soaks and by whether she's progressively gaining weight. If you feel your milk supply is short, pump both breasts after nursing two or three times a day—not after every feeding. Store any pumped milk that your baby doesn't need immediately. Building up a supply of stored milk will allow other people (i.e. dad) to feed the baby and offer you some freedom. With pumping three to four times per day your milk supply should increase within three to five days. If you find after doing so, you're still having trouble with supply, consult a lactation specialist. There's nothing wrong with supplementing breast-feeding with formula.

If you feel your milk supply is "excessive" (this is rare), enjoy the bounty. Pump three to four times per day after feedings and build up an arsenal of stored milk.

Introducing a Bottle: Feeding the Baby Pumped Milk or Formula

As stated above, as long as artificial nipples and pacifiers are introduced prior to one month of age, most babies will easily switch between the real nipple, a bottle nipple, or a pacifier.

Bottle nipples seem to go through frequent trendy re-designs. Some claim to be endorsed by pediatricians or dentists. Realistically, most nipples are supple enough that they'll conform to whatever shape your baby's tongue and palate make while nursing.

The size of the nipple opening seems to be more important to babies than the shape of an artificial nipple. Too small and the slow flow frustrates the baby. Too large and the flow may flood the baby's mouth too quickly for her to swallow. Experiment with different artificial nipples to see which your baby prefers.

Storing pumped milk and supplementing

You can store pumped milk in the refrigerator for one week or in the freezer for one month. Use stored milk before it "expires", not so much because the milk "goes bad", but because breast milk changes over time and what your baby needed at six weeks of age may not be what he needs at four months of age.

If you're working you may not be able to keep up with the baby's demand. It's *okay*. Pump and feed him what you can, nurse when you're home from work, and supplement with a formula recommended by your pediatrician or lactation specialist.

When I went back to work after delivery, my stored milk supply dwindled and the amount I pumped during the day couldn't match my baby's needs. So we supplemented. I breast-fed at night, pumped as much as possible during the day for my husband to feed the baby the following day. Our babies also got one to three bottles of formula per day. Both babies weaned from the breast at ten months. By then they were also eating solid food. They both wound up fat, healthy, and smart.

Formula Feeding

I'm sure you've heard the benefits of breast-feeding from many sources: the immunity protection, the bonding possibilities. Some experts even make the claim that breast fed babies are smarter. I doubt there's much truth to the latter, unless you're looking at second or third world countries where quality of formula may be very low. The World Health Organization sets standards for human milk substitutes, but these may or may not be followed, depending on the country's governmental regulation of its formula-producing industry. First-world formula is quality stuff.

If you decide not to breast-feed don't worry about it and don't feel guilty. Millions of children, including myself, were formula-fed from the 1950's through the 1980's when breastfeeding was "out of style". Well, I never got sick as a child, was always at the top of my class and went to medical school. Formula appeared to do me and millions of others in my generation no harm.

You may simply not be interested in breast-feeding. Or you may have trouble with supply due to many reasons: premature delivery, nipple problems, and previous breast surgery, among others. Don't worry or stress over it.

The biggest benefits of breast-feeding are the skin-to-skin contact with the baby and the immune proteins in breast milk. Formula is good but it cannot duplicate these two things unless you formula-feed with the baby skin-to-skin as though he were on the breast. This can be awkward, but on the up side, it gives dad the opportunity to "breast-feed".

In our experience the biggest drawback to formula was its preparation and expense: you have to heat the water just so and add the formula. We had a bottle heater to heat both breast milk and formula, but often the baby waited on it (screaming the whole time). Plus a can of powdered formula cost eleven dollars when our kids were babies. In comparison, breast milk is free, prepackaged at just the right temperature, no mess, and no fuss.

If you are willing to and can breast-feed I recommend doing so simply for its cost (free) and lack of fussy preparation, in addition to the health benefits for you and the baby. In the long run even a high quality breast pump such as a Medela Pump-N-Style is cheaper than the cans and cans of formula you'll need to purchase if you formula-feed exclusively.

Options to deal with prematurity or nipple problems is to forego the actual breast-feeding and simply pump your milk and feed the baby pumped breast milk. Babies do fine with this method.

Nipple Problems

Sore or cracked nipples are nearly universal, especially for first-time moms. These problems can be traced back to latch-on technique. I cannot stress enough the importance of the baby approaching the nipple with a wide open

> **Nipple soreness is usually due to latch on technique and can be alleviated by adjusting the latch on.**

mouth. When the baby is properly latched on, his lips contact the areola, and pressure of the nipple on his palate provokes proper tongue motion and suckling technique.

For almost everyone, there's a "break in" period of one to two weeks as you and the baby get the hang of the latch-on. Every baby's different. Your second or third child may be a completely different type of suckler than your first child. During the break-in period most people have sore nipples and areolas. Eventually these will "toughen up". This and the baby becoming a more proficient nurser will ultimately relieve nipple and areola soreness.

Treatments for sore nipples include applying Lansinoh, Lanolin, or some other nipple ointment after feeding. You don't have to wipe this off between feedings. Nipple ointments designed for human lactation are non-toxic to the baby. You can also wear plastic nipple protectors between feedings so your bra or shirt isn't further abrading your sore nipples.

Cracked nipples may require more care and attention. Cracked nipples are usually a result of the baby "chewing" his way onto the nipple, rather than latching on with a wide open mouth. Some babies have a short "frenulum"—a strand of tissue attaching the underside of the tongue to the floor of the mouth. A short frenulum limits the baby from drawing the nipple against the palate and causes the baby to exert more friction on the nipple during suckling. If you've evaluated your latch-on technique and the baby seems to be latching on with a wide open mouth, but you still have cracked, sore nipples, consult your pediatrician and/or a lactation specialist. A lactation specialist can help you identify if the problems is due to latch-on technique or to anatomic factors relating to your baby's mouth and your nipples. A pediatrician can snip a short frenulum with no ill effects to the baby, and it may resolve the latch-on problem by allowing the baby greater tongue mobility.

Sometimes your nipples become so sore or cracked the only solution is to take a short break from breast-feeding. In this situation, pump your milk with a double electric pump, and feed your baby the pumped breast milk via a bottle. Use nipple protectors between your nipples and bra for a few days. Apply nipple ointment liberally. Most cracked nipples will heal adequately with two days' "rest" from the baby, to re-initiate latch-on.

You can use nipple shields to manage flat, inverted or cracked nipples. Nipple shields are silicone nipple-areola covering devices that allow the baby to latch on and draw out your nipple into the tip of the shield. Nipple shields are usually only necessary for a few days during which the nipple problem resolves. Consult a lactation specialist or post-partum nurse to determine if you'd benefit from nipple shields, and be instructed in their use.

Mastitis

Mastitis is a serious infection of the breast that responds rapidly to antibiotics, when diagnosed properly. Mastitis can occur at any time during lactation, even months into it. Often the first symptoms of mastitis have nothing to do with your breasts: You may feel suddenly tired, with body aches, and a fever, like you have the flu. You may or may not have a sore and red patch on one of your breasts. Notify your health care provider immediately because mastitis responds quickly to antibiotics. However, without rapid intervention you can become very ill and may need hospitalization for intravenous antibiotics.

The risk of mastitis can be minimized with good attention to nipple care and minimizing breast engorgement. Continue breast-feeding or pumping through mastitis because if you don't the ensuing engorgement can worsen the problem.

Suppression of Milk Supply

You may choose not to breast-feed for a number of reasons: You just don't feel like it; you're giving your baby up for adoption; you're having problems with milk supply; you've had breast surgery, or a myriad of others.

If it's a supply problem or previous breast surgery, you probably won't need to take action to suppress your milk supply.

However if you have normal milk supply and want to suppress lactation there are a number of methods. You may need to pump occasionally to relieve pain of engorgement but try not to pump more than once daily, or you'll stimulate milk supply to increase. Use a wimpy hand pump rather than a double electric pump; and pump only enough to relieve engorgement—do not completely empty the breast. Over a few days the unemptied breast will send a signal to your brain to shut down the lactation machinery and your milk will dry up.

You can also apply cold ice packs or cold cabbage leaves (they conform to breast shape). The cold constricts breast blood vessels and thereby reduces milk production. It also relieves pain from engorgement.

Estrogen-containing birth control pills can suppress your milk supply but these take longer to act and are better for maintaining a suppressed milk supply than to induce suppression of milk supply.

In the "old days" a medication, bromocriptine or Parlodel, was prescribed to suppress lactation. However, this practice has fallen by the wayside due to side effects of this medication such as headache, nausea, and vomiting. The non-pharmaceutical methods for lactation suppression are quite effective.

Neonatal Jaundice

Neonatal jaundice is a common finding in newborns and is revealed as a bronzing of the skin due to the newborn's inability to metabolize a substance called bilirubin. Bilirubin is a breakdown product of red blood cells that is normally processed in the liver. Preterm infants are at greatest risk for jaundice, but the phenomenon can occur in term infants as well.

Neonatal jaundice often resolves spontaneously as the infant becomes proficient at breast-feeding, your milk comes in, and his liver matures. High bilirubin levels (>25mg/dL) were at one time thought to be associated with neurologic problems and seizures. However, later research has called this relationship into question. Nevertheless, if your baby remains jaundiced, his bilirubin levels will be monitored and he'll be treated with blue light phototherapy if the levels fail to fall spontaneously.

Blue light phototherapy breaks bilirubin in the skin down to water soluble molecules that can be excreted by the kidneys. It is administered either by overhead "bili lights" or via a "bili blanket". Sunlight accomplishes the same end result, but blue light phototherapy avoids the risk of sunburn.

Because phototherapy converts bilirubin to water-soluble molecules, it is very important your infant remain well hydrated so he can excrete these byproducts in the urine. Breast-feed frequently (every two to three hours) and supplement if necessary to keep your infant well hydrated. If your baby has jaundice treatment will be guided by your pediatrician.

Baby Blues and Post-Partum Depression: Why They Occur and How to Tell the Difference: How to Know When you Need Help

A momentous hormonal shift occurs in the first two weeks post-partum.

Imagine this: At the end of pregnancy your brain is awash in a sea of progesterone and estrogen. Your endorphin levels (the body's "happy molecules") are high because, as you learned in chapters three and four, estrogen and progesterone

> **Baby blues and post partum depression are triggered by the tremendous drop in hormones (estrogen and progesterone) after childbirth.**

increase your innate endorphin levels. Moreover, progesterone is an anxiolytic—it sort of acts like valium in calming the nerves and contributing to a sensation of "mellowness".

Now this: After the baby and placenta come out of your body, your estrogen and progesterone levels plummet. Think of it as falling off a cliff. Moreover, your milk hormone, prolactin increases dramatically in the first few days. Prolactin eventually suppresses your estrogen and progesterone levels close to those of a menopausal woman. Luckily, prolactin and breast-feeding also stimulate the innate endorphins; otherwise, all pregnant women would be deeply depressed.

There's a two week window in the post-partum period, between delivery of the baby and onset of consistently high prolactin levels, when you're likely to experience maximum "baby blues". Baby blues are like the worst case of PMS you've ever had: You're on an emotional roller coaster because your endorphin levels are all over the place. One minute you're blissfully happy with your perfect newborn;

the next you're weeping uncontrollably. The onset of baby blues often corresponds to the Night of Inconsolable Crying or to breast-feeding difficulties.

Remember this: baby blues are transitional and you can ride them out. Baby blues respond to a change in scenery, sleep, and some help from your spouse. If you're in a deep well of crying go for a thirty minute brisk walk. The physical activity and fresh air will instantly brighten your mood. Don't over-extend. Lots of company in the first week postpartum can be stressful. Too many visitors? Just Say No (thank you).

Eighty-five percent of women experience baby blues; ten to fifteen percent go on to have post-partum depression. Baby blues typically resolve within six weeks post-partum.; whereas post-partum depression can begin anytime in the first year after delivery.

Postpartum depression is characterized by:

- ➢ Feelings of Constant or Recurring Anxiety
- ➢ Loss of Control
- ➢ Loneliness, Dysphoria (feelings of gloom)
- ➢ Self-Doubt
- ➢ Feeling inadequate as a parent; unrealistic expectations of parenthood
- ➢ Feelings of impending doom such as loss of or harm to a loved one
- ➢ Feeling emotionally detached from the baby
- ➢ Lack of motivation to care for yourself and/or the baby
- ➢ Thoughts of harming yourself or the baby

Physical symptoms often accompany the emotional side of postpartum depression. These include:

- ➢ Sleep disorders: insomnia and/or inability to get out of bed in the morning
- ➢ Fatigue
- ➢ Appetite changes: Lack of appetite or overeating for comfort
- ➢ Stomach upset, nausea, indigestion, diarrhea
- ➢ Decrease in milk supply

Risk factors for postpartum depression include:

- ➢ History in yourself or a family member of depression or bipolar disorder
- ➢ Financial stressors

➤ Housing stressors
➤ Marital stressors
➤ Depression during pregnancy
➤ Low self-esteem
➤ Physical isolation (being home alone all day with the baby)

Contact your health care provider if you feel you're experiencing postpartum depression. Postpartum depression can be serious but it responds to changes in your family support structure, exercise, counseling, and antidepressants.

Feelings of Detachment

It is not unusual for new moms and dads to undergo brief periods of detachment. From time to time you may wonder, "What on earth have we done?" Being a new parent can cause you to relive some of the experiences of your childhood and being parented by your parents. These may be positive or negative. Some of you may want to be completely different parents than your own because of negative feelings about your childhood. Others of you may feel like there's no way you'll live up to create the childhood and home environment your parents established for you. You may at times feel overwhelmed with the responsibility of being a parent, and with a feeling of being tied down "forever".

Anxiety about parenthood and feelings of detachment can be managed by breaking them down into their component elements and addressing each one. If you fear not being an adequate parent, what are the specifics of that fear? Write down the details that come to mind then address each one individually. Write down your solutions or avenues to improvement. You may be able to do this with your spouse; you may not, depending on your relationship. At any rate, you've brought this life into the world and it's up to you and only you to be the best mother or father you can for that baby.

Sleep deprivation and exhaustion can exaggerate any negative emotions you experience and decrease your coping skills. Strategies to minimize fatigue include sleeping when the baby sleeps; taking "shifts" for feed-

> **Sleep deprivation can exacerbate any negative emotions experienced following childbirth.**

ings and diaper changings, and taking regularly scheduled "breaks" from the baby. If you're lucky enough to have a trusted relative live close enough to watch the baby so you both can go out together. If not, you can spell one another from time to time. Check in with yourself and with your spouse on a regular basis.

Rehabilitating Your Pelvic Floor

If you don't want the bad news, skip this section and go on to the next one addressing Kegel Exercises. There's no doubt about it. Pregnancy changes your bottom. The weight of the baby for nine months on your pelvic floor muscles and nerves weakens of those nerves through pressure. Recent electromyographic research (a technique used to measure muscle strength and neuromuscular activity) on the pelvic floor has shown that twenty percent of the "damage" to the pelvic floor occurs throughout pregnancy. This "damage" is defined as a decrease in muscle strength and in neuromuscular activity. Another twenty-five percent occurs with vaginal delivery. Fifteen percent is lost with vaginal labor that ultimately ends in a C-section. C-section for a dysfunctional labor is minimally protective of the pelvic floor.

- **20% of the "damage" to the pelvic floor occurs throughout pregnancy**
- **Another 25% occurs with vaginal delivery**
- **15% is lost with vaginal labor that ultimately ends in a C-section**

C-section without labor is only partially protective of the pelvic floor because twenty-five percent of the loss of muscle strength has already occurred during pregnancy. I perform plenty of incontinence and pelvic reconstruction surgeries for women who had all their babies via C-section.

Vaginal delivery changes the axis and caliber of the vagina. Before you're ever pregnant, as you're standing, the long axis of the vagina is horizontal or parallel to the ground (zero degrees). After a vaginal delivery, the long axis of the vagina points downward anywhere from ten to ninety degrees, depending on how many babies you've borne, what your deliveries were like, and your age. This change in axis is due to a stretching of the levator muscles (reviewed in Chapter Six) and to stretching of the pudendal nerve that innervates these muscles. Stretching of a nerve causes it to not function as well—it doesn't fire with the same frequency or intensity. Since firing of nerves stimulates growth of muscle size, less nerve firing means smaller muscle fibers which translate to weaker muscles.

Moreover, a vaginal birth enlarges the "genital hiatus". The genital hiatus encompasses the natural perforations in the levator ani muscles made by the vagina, urethra, and rectum. When a full term baby comes through that space, it enlarges the canals in these muscles through which these organs pass.

The combination of the changes in vaginal axis and the enlargement of the genital hiatus (the droopy loosey vagina) contribute to a problem known as "pelvic organ prolapse". This is a situation in which the uterus can slide down the vagina (uterine prolapse); the bladder can "fall" into the vagina (a cystocele); and the rectum can "pooch" into the vagina (a rectocele).

Symptoms of pelvic organ prolapse (POP) can occur immediately or can gradually develop or worsen over time. These includes unintentional loss of urine (urinary incontinence), unintentional loss of gas (flatus incontinence), trapping of air in the vagina followed by its forced expulsion with movement or change in position (vaginal "farts"), and a sensation something's "falling out" of the vagina (uterine prolapse). Over years POP can result in low back pain from the uterine ligaments pulling on the lower spine, unintentional loss of stool (incontinence of stool) and digital defecation—a situation where the muscular wall between the rectum and vagina becomes so weak you need to place a finger in the vagina to support the rectum so hard stool can exit the anus.

Sounds awful, doesn't it? Reason enough to just forget the whole baby thing. Don't despair, **you can prevent and/or correct this**.

Kegels to the Rescue!

You can reverse the damage caused to your pelvic nerves and muscles with Kegel Exercises. As soon as your bottom stops feeling tender from delivery, start your Kegels.

How to do Kegels: Contract the muscles inside the vagina as though you're going to stop your urine stream or pinch off a bowel movement. Hold this contraction for three to five seconds. Repeat ten times. Do not push down with your abdominal muscles. Instead visualize your pelvic muscles as a bowl at the bottom of your pelvis. You want to squeeze that bowl closed like the leaves of the shutter of a camera. To be certain you've got the right muscles, lie down on your back and place two fingers in your vagina. When doing a Kegel contraction you should feel the vagina close down around your fingers. Hold that contraction for three to five seconds. If you don't "get it" at first, keep trying until you get it right. Trust me—it'll do you a world of good in the long run and may even improve your sex life.

When to do Kegels: Do a set of ten (10) Kegels every time you change diapers and begin them as soon as soreness from delivery has resolved. Given your baby will go through ten to twelve diapers per day; you'll be doing at least 100 to 120 Kegels per day if you adhere to this schedule. Once your baby's outgrown diapers, do Kegels every time the phone rings; when you're talking on the phone; during commercials when watching television; and at stoplights when driving. Kegel when you're cooking. Kegel when you're cleaning. Kegel when you're waiting in line at the grocery store. Kegel during sex. Kegel 'til the cows come home.

When *not* to do Kegels: Do not intentionally interrupt your urine stream or a bowl movement to do a Kegel. This can cause "neuromuscular confusion" and lead to urinary urgency or other dysfunction of the urine and bowels.

How do Kegels work? Like any exercise, Kegels increase the size of the muscle fibers. They also stimulate blood flow to the muscles and nerves of the pelvis. They can reverse damage to your pudendal nerve through the positive feedback from the intentional muscle contraction. Kegels can narrow the caliber of your vagina to near-pre-pregnancy levels. They can reverse the dropping of the vaginal axis. They can improve or resolve incontinence and improve sexual function.

Sex After Baby

You can have sex six weeks after a vaginal birth or C-section. The reason for waiting six weeks is to allow the cervix to fully close. This will prevent the mechanical action of sex from moving vaginal bacteria into the uterus and causing a uterine infection.

Just because you *can* have sex at six weeks does not mean you will *want* to. Most women experience a decrease in sex drive after baby due to a number of factors: Fatigue, lactation being a "hypoestrogenized state", vaginal dryness and pain, and feeling emotionally spent by the baby.

Fatigue: Face it. You're up every few hours the first six weeks with the baby. You're giving her all you've got. You're learning how to be a parent. And you just plain don't have the energy for anything else, much less sex. Fatigue impacts both parents, not just mom. You may even attempt sex, but get interrupted by a crying baby. While the desire to view your husband as merely the sperm contributor may be high at this time, try to find a way to re-establish the marital, not just the parental bonds. This may mean having a relative or friend babysit while you go out on a "date". The date may not even lead to sex—don't expect it to or the pressure will kill it. The most you can expect from it is remembering why you married your spouse and embarked on this journey of parenthood; the least is an interesting conversation about the infinite varieties of baby poop.

Lactation is a Hypoestrogenized State—Reduces Sex Drive: Lactation has similar hormonal effects as menopause. The milk-producing hormone (prolactin) suppresses your estrogen, progesterone, and testosterone levels to a near-menopausal level. Estrogen and testosterone normally stimulate your sex drive, and their suppression can seriously dampen your sex drive. During lactation you may even experience night sweats, hot flashes, and vaginal dryness. Sounds like menopause—doesn't it?

Vaginal Dryness: Due to lack of estrogen, over a few months the vaginal skin can become less lubricated and thin out. This can cause pain with intercourse—it feels like sandpaper. Moreover, you may have scar tissue from a repair that protests the friction of intercourse. Vaginal dryness can be treated with over-the-counter lubricants such as Replens, K-Y, and Astroglide; or a prescription estrogen vaginal cream. Consult your health care provider if you have persistent vaginal discomfort not relieved with over-the-counter preparations.

Spending It All on Baby: Even if you're not breast-feeding, you're spending all your emotional and physical energy on Baby. He's a new person—you want to get to know him. He's vulnerable and needy. It's a twenty-four-seven job attending to his bodily functions—feeding, comfort, peeing and pooping. It's all you can do to take care of him, much less attend to someone else's needs like sex. After all you can hardly even get a daily shower in because you're constantly attending to the baby and when you're not, you're asleep. If you can, find a way to take time out, both for just yourself, and for you and your spouse. Many husbands understand of the lack of sex drive because they see how exhausted you are and they're exhausted themselves. However, it doesn't hurt to make the effort to re-establish marital intimacy, even if it's only cuddling.

Sex Drive Rebounds

As your baby gets older, is weaned from lactation, and you get more sleep, your hormone levels will return to normal. However, you may or may not ever have the same sex drive you had pre-pregnancy. Or in some cases you may have even more sex drive. You may notice your sex drive becomes more pronouncedly cyclic—peaking after your menses and around ovulation and dropping after ovulation before onset of menses. You can tell when you're ovulating by the time in your cycle (usually day twelve to fourteen) and the production of a clear mucous discharge. Sex drive tends to be highest between days six and fourteen of the menstrual cycle (also corresponds to the greatest chances for pregnancy).

Anatomic Changes Affect Sex: What to Do

Remember all that stuff you read or skipped over under "Rehabilitating Your Pelvic Floor"? Well sex after baby may feel different due to these changes. You may feel "looser" and may actually have loss of sensation in areas which previously had a significant amount of sensation.

The key to restoring your sex life is kegel, kegel, kegel. Through kegeling you'll refurbish your anatomy to as normal as possible, improve the blood flow and nerve sensation to the pelvic muscles, and may even have a better sex life compared to before pregnancy.

If you have specific, localized pain, especially at the site of a tear, consult your health care provider. This problem can be addressed with prescription estrogen cream, but sometimes needs revision of a repair to completely relieve the discomfort.

Mile Markers: Six Weeks and Twelve Weeks

The first few weeks of parenthood may devolve into a flurry of feedings, diaper changing's, middle-of-the-night crying sessions (for both you and the baby). You may wonder, will life ever be "normal" again? No it won't; but eventually it'll be better than normal as you watch your child grow and evolve into a full-fledged person.

Moreover, infants under six weeks of age aren't very interactive. When awake they just look about and take it all in. You may wonder, "Is this all?"

Six weeks is a major milestone. By six weeks your infant will have head control; he may even begin to smile, giggle, and become more responsive to your attempts to engage his attention. He'll also be a proficient nurser, be a better sleeper, and have a more consistent schedule. You'll begin to feel like he's giving something back to you for all the effort you've put into him. He'll seem less like a bottomless pit of neediness.

Many of your breast issues will be resolved by six weeks. You'll be proficient at latch-on. Nipple soreness will have improved. You'll be familiar with the let-down reflex and sensations associated with this.

In those wee hours of the night when you're feeding your baby or walking him around the house during a bout of inconsolable crying, repeat to yourself: "Six weeks, six weeks." Once you make it through the first six weeks life improves.

Twelve weeks is another major hurdle. If you have a "colicky" baby, the problem usually resolves or significantly decreases by twelve weeks of age. Whatever is behind "colic"—intestinal gas, immature digestive system, or just being an infant, seems to sort itself out by twelve weeks of age.

By twelve weeks your infant has "personality" and gives you back all you put into him and more. The love between you grows and you feel less like a milk machine or cow, and more like a mom.

If you can survive the first six weeks, you'll make it to twelve. If you survive the first three months, you'll get to one year. At six months your baby will be sitting upright, babbling, and playing. By one year he'll be walking (or running). This all seems to drag by while you're in the midst of it, but when you're child is entering kindergarten or going off to middle school, you'll barely remember it and time will have seemed to evaporate. Cherish every moment.

Some Nuts and Bolts of Infant Care

Head Control

At birth your baby's nervous system is still very immature. She's not coordinated and usually can't even hold up her head. Head control and muscle coordination develop as her nerves become myelinated (are sheathed with the layer of insulation that speeds nerve signals). The fact that you have to support her head may make you tentative and anxious about newborn care. This is normal. As she matures, she gains head control by six weeks of age, sometimes sooner.

Car Seat

The most important piece of baby equipment is your car seat. Many hospitals require in their criteria for discharge, that you possess and demonstrate proper use of a car seat. Because the baby initially lacks head control you may want to use rolled up baby blankets or a preformed head support while the baby is in the car seat for the first six weeks.

Pediatrician Visits

Unless the baby has problems with jaundice, breast-feeding, or weight gain, the first pediatrician visit will usually be at two weeks of age. The pediatrician will address normal development with you, weight gain, and vaccination intervals. Write down your questions for the pediatrician ahead of time so you make sure they're addressed at the visit.

Circumcision

In the "old days" circumcision used to be performed on male infants before they left the hospital. It has become common practice to defer circumcision until two weeks of age; and now it is done in the pediatrician's office or at a "brisque", depending on your religious affiliation. The pediatrician usually uses local anesthetic for the circumcision, another advance in the procedure. Circumcision is not a medically necessary procedure and your pediatrician will address the pros and cons with you.

Preventing SIDS: Back to Sleep and No Smoking

Sudden Infant Death Syndrome (SIDS) affects 55/100,000 infants annually under age one year and can be reduced by two major interventions: Placing the baby on his back when laying him down to sleep and not smoking in the house or at all.

SIDS is most common between two and four months of age. Additional measures you can take to protect your baby against SIDS are 1) use a firm mattress; 2) do not surround the baby with soft toys and pillows in his crib or bassinet; and 3) if you're using a nanny or infant care provider, communicate with them the measures they'll take to reduce the risk of SIDS. Make sure they understand the principle of laying the baby on his back when placing him down to sleep. If he's later found sleeping on his stomach, you or your child care provider should reposition him so he's on his back.

Smoking and use of illicit drugs is associated with a higher incidence of SIDS. If you or your spouse haven't already quit during pregnancy, it's time to quit now. If you need help quitting there are many non-prescription and prescription smoking cessation aids on the market. Additional strategies to help you quit smoking include: 1) Set a quit date; 2) Find something else to do with your hands and mouth (e.g. chew gum); 3) Avoid socializing with smokers, or ask them not to smoke in your presence because you're trying to quit. 4) Join a smoking cessation support group which can usually be found through your local hospital or health care provider.

If you just can't quit, at least refrain from smoking in the house. Minimize the particulates in your home by cleaning the carpets, washing curtains and walls, and using an air filter in the baby's room to capture smoke and other particles.

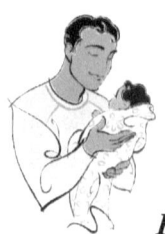

For Dads: Why the Breasts May Be Off-Limits

Wow! You're wife's breast-feeding and you've hit the jackpot. Now she has triple D ultra humungous Playboy bunny breasts. Unfortunately they come equipped with an alarm that shouts, "Please step away from the breasts!" as soon as you're in the vicinity.

While nursing your wife often thinks of her breasts as merely for feeding the baby. They are sore and tender at first. It's fine for the baby to touch them because they're for him. But as for you: Well, you might want to forget it for a while. She may feel like she just can't stand one more person pawing at her breasts. She's getting more than enough breast contact from the baby and her breasts may temporarily cease to be sexual.

Moreover, when you do touch them she may begin leaking. This isn't really pleasant and can actually be somewhat annoying, depending on the person. Each woman is different and some are more sexually turned on by breast contact while lactating than others. Try not to be disappointed or take it personally if your wife is one of the many who is not. Like all things, this too shall pass.

Chapter 10

The Leading Man—Knight in Shining Armor

"Shock and Awe"

For many men the time during the first half of their wife's pregnancy the baby seems like an abstract thing. It starts to feel more real when her belly is noticeably large and you can feel the baby move. My husband and my clients' fathers-to-be universally describe that moment as "really cool".

The arrival of the baby is altogether different. Feelings range from excitement to wonder, a sensation of spirituality; and being overwhelmed, anxious, and not ready. Many men simultaneously experience all these emotions to varying degrees.

> **Having the baby is like receiving the diploma without attending school.**

While your wife has had nine months to "take care of" and adapt to this new person in your life; the actual presence of the baby for dads is like receiving the diploma without having gone to school. You're expected to know what to do with it and with little physical training other than some generalities discussed in prenatal classes. Your reaction and sense of preparation may have a great deal to do with your age and maturity level; and whether the pregnancy was planned.

The arrival of your child puts you in touch with your own mortality and the circle of life. You see first-hand just how fragile and resilient life can be.

Fatherhood: Long-Term Commitment, Not a Rite of Passage

Most modern men realize human babies require two parents to raise them and are eager to take part in the care of their newborn. A few seem to view parenthood from the "macho" perspective as a rite of passage or a confirmation of manhood. This only hurts your heir and your woman.

Now that you've helped create this new person you are responsible for seeing them have a healthy, stable, secure life. You're not fifty percent responsible. You are one hundred percent responsible. Your marriage will be stronger and more fun if you take an active role in parenting, anticipate your wife's needs, and try to make her life easier. She has an exhausting job just breast-feeding a baby. That takes a lot out of a person—physically and emotionally. You can be the knight in shining armor, the hero, for your wife and your child by changing diapers, giving the baby a bath, cleaning the house, and cooking. You may have been at work all day; but so has your wife—she's been constantly "in demand" taking care of a very helpless living thing.

Neither of you have slept well in weeks, but your wife is the one getting up every two hours at night for feedings—at least initially.

Conquering Fear

Both parents experience moments (or days) of dread and anxiety. There are several things to keep in mind and techniques to manage fear and anxiety.

The first thing to realize it is safe to hold the baby. He won't break; you just need to be aware of supporting his head because most babies lack head control until six weeks of age.

Gain confidence through mastery of the details. Hold the baby. He will recognize your voice, your touch, and your face from very early on. Bathe him. Change his diaper. Learn how to use a bottle warmer and give him a bottle. Become an expert belcher (I know from experience boys undergo intensive belch training during the sixth grade and are masters of the process mere weeks into the school year;

Conquering Fear:
- **It's safe to hold the baby— in fact he enjoys your touch.**
- **Gain overall confidence through mastery of the details.**
- **Remind yourself each stage is temporary.**

that training stays with you forever). At about six months of age babies begin to take solid food. Learn what your baby enjoys and take part in feeding him.

Early parenthood defines taking life "day by day". Remember every stage is temporary. Enjoy the good parts of each stage and understand the difficult parts will pass. If you make it through the first day, you'll make it through the first week. If you survive the first week, you can make it to six weeks. Six weeks … three months. Three months … six months. Six months … one year.

How to be the Knight in Shining Armor

During pregnancy the most you can do to help is clean the house, and help cook; fetch ice cream and other late-night craving items. You can attend important visits such as the first visit, the twenty week visit or ultrasound and one of the weekly visits in the last month. Prenatal classes are also an opportunity to learn about your baby, labor, and your wife.

During labor just being there and being supportive of your wife's choices is crucial. She may not be the nicest person in labor—don't take it personal; labor hurts. Remain calm if she says "I hate you" and her head spins and out comes green vomit. It's only temporary. It's the pain speaking, not her.

The first six weeks is an opportunity for you to really shine and make your wife fall more deeply in love with you. Your actions in the first six weeks can also begin to develop seeds of disappointment and resentment. She will probably suppress her disappointment or sublimate it in denial. Keep in touch; talk to her—ask her how she's feeling. It's in both your interests—your emotional health, your physical health, your financial health and your baby's well-being—to be a good father.

You Will Be Ignored—It's Nothing Personal

The baby will consume your wife's attention and energy. You may feel like an afterthought in her day. This is normal and it also will pass; especially if you engage yourself in being a parent and in helping out. Your wife's romantic interest is directly proportional to the energy you put into helping with the baby and keeping the house running. It is simple math: The more housework you do, the more sex you get. There really is a strong correlation. If your wife's too tired to have sex, maybe it's because she's being overworked because you aren't taking care of the house.

If you view taking care of the house as your number one priority during the first six weeks of parenthood, while your wife is learning how to breast-feed and coping with hormone changes, baby blues or postpartum depression, you will earn many "husband points". The more husband points you earn, the more likely you'll get sex down the road and the more likely your marriage will be successful overall. Don't be afraid to point out to your wife, "Look what I did: vacuumed, cleaned the bathrooms, cooked dinner, etc." A word of caution: Do not brag about your housekeeping prowess to the point of annoyance.

> **Make the most of the time your wife is focused on the baby to rack up husband points in the favor bank. You will be able to cash them in later.**

There are too many children growing up in single parent homes.

They will survive. I grew up in one and I survived. But it is extremely difficult for the child and the single parent. Being the child of divorced parents can lead to life-long insecurities and predispose people to anxiety and depression. Many children of divorced parents develop fears of abandonment that impact their relationships for the rest of their lives. Children feel much more stable in two-parent households. You have the power to completely affect another person's life; use it wisely and with discretion.

You can really solidify your marriage bonds by being a great dad, especially during the difficult first six weeks.

Hint: For the *exceedingly rare* few of you who don't know, the "on" switch for the vacuum is usually located somewhere on the handle. It's a tool—men are supposed to love tools—aren't they? Familiarize yourself with it and put it to use on at least a weekly basis.

Transform Setbacks into Opportunities

Setbacks are inevitable. There will be moments, days, and weeks that rattle your confidence and make you feel completely inept. Babies will have nights when they don't sleep and are inconsolable. Accept this as inevitable. You'll get past it and things will be better in a day or two.

Parenthood is a quantum leap in responsibility but you can use this as an opportunity for growth. Change your mind set. You don't have to do things the same old way. You may discover talents you never knew you possessed—awaken your unrealized potential.

Anticipate your wife's and your baby's needs. Be proactive about helping. Create a nice home for your family. Your needs are now secondary—if you can't play poker or watch the ball game because the baby needs attending to or your wife needs a respite, oh well. There will be other games. Suck it up and above all: No Whining.

Ambiguity

All parents experience moments of ambiguity. They're not sure they really love this new being—she's so needy and demanding. How can a person satisfy someone who at times seems impossible to please? Hopefully you and your wife won't be struck with simultaneous bouts of ambiguity. If one person is "up" it's easier for them to help the other person who's "down". You and your wife may frequently switch roles.

A father may have a greater degree of resentment toward the baby than the mother because he's being ignored. All her time is the baby's; her breasts are off limits ("they're for the baby") and she does not want to have sex.

Breasts

Wow look at those hooters! She's got the biggest, plumpest breasts you've ever seen outside of a girly mag. But wait—you can look but chances are she doesn't want you to touch. Frankly, the baby's

> **Lactating breasts are often sore; she may be annoyed if you touch them.**

been on them all day and night and she's just sick of feeling like a cow. Her breasts may be tender if engorged, her nipples may be cracked; and she may have some pain related to breast-feeding.

Touching her breasts or having sex may lead to milk let-down and leaking. She may or may not be "turned on" by you sucking her nipples like the baby. Some women find that exciting; others are repulsed. Don't hesitate to ask her how she feels. Her feelings may change from day-to-day or week to week so it doesn't hurt to periodically "check in".

Unfortunately the lactating breasts do not stay the same size, shape or plumpness, after weaning. Many women are very self conscious about this. They may not want to have sex after weaning because they're embarrassed about their breasts and other aspects of their post-baby bodies (see below). If you care about these things you may ask yourself is this an important thing to care about or is it not. Have frank discussions with your wife. If she's self-conscious about her body, the fastest way you can get your sex life back after baby is to make her feel reassured about her body. Recognize most women retain an extra five to ten pounds during the six months or year of breast-feeding. Don't pressure her to look like her pre-pregnancy self by six weeks after the baby arrives.

Sex After Baby—Patience—She's Not There Yet

Women experience major physical and emotional changes during pregnancy, birth, and post partum.

Physically, her body has been stretched and is often different after pregnancy. Her bottom may hurt for weeks, especially if she had a bad tear. Breast-feeding is a low-estrogen state so she may experience vaginal dryness, pain with intercourse, and hot flashes. Good sex during this time will require extra foreplay and extra lubrication.

Pregnancy and birth stretches the vaginal nerves, muscles, and skin. It normally takes a minimum of six weeks—sometimes three months or more—to regain vaginal muscle control, and control over bladder and bowel function. Your wife may "fart" uncontrollably. Don't be shocked or grossed out—it's just a fact of life. The nerve sensation and muscle tone just isn't there for self control.

You should avoid intercourse for six weeks after birth because the cervix remains open for six weeks and the risk of serious uterus infection increases with intercourse. And trust me ... this is not the time to ask her for a blow job unless you want to invite the nearest sharp implement to have a close encounter eye socket.

Your wife's sexual organs change with pregnancy and childbirth. She may feel "looser". This eventually corrects itself, especially if your wife does her kegel exercises—ten times during every diaper changing beginning the day after delivery.

How to Get Her Interested Again

Housework, date nights, thoughtful gifts. The most important things you can do are keep a neat house cook meals before everyone is starving and grumpy. If your wife is irritable and it's been at least two hours since she's eaten—make her a snack. Even if she says no, she'll eat it anyway.

Your wife and you may be reluctant to spend any time away from the baby during the first six weeks. However, if you can arrange a date with reliable child care—grasp the opportunity! It's a chance to get back in touch with the love you feel for each other that led you to create this child in the first place.

Work and Family Balance; Consistency

It is important to discuss post-baby roles during pregnancy, long before the baby is born. Most households have two earners essential to financial viability. If your wife has the higher paying job, it may make sense for you to stay home with the kid(s) unless you both can make enough to cover day care so it's not a strain on the family budget.

Be flexible. Parental roles change throughout raising children. Do not undermine or contradict each other. Try to maintain consistency in what you tell your children, and the boundaries you set for them. Don't disparage each other, especially in front of the children. Your children love you both and you will never get them "on your side". Children are confused by parents' negative comments towards each other—just don't do it.

How to Recognize Postpartum Depression

After delivery your wife's hormones drop from the stratosphere to well below the sub-basement. Read chapter three again if you don't recall the intense impact of hormones on the brain.

Rapid drops in estrogen and progesterone can precipitate crying spells, moodiness, "baby blues" and outright depression. Eighty percent of women get baby blues. Weepiness may appear irrationally and without warning; such as at sentimental things like television commercials.

As the milk-production hormones rise, they suppress your wife's estrogen and progesterone levels. By six weeks after delivery these levels may approach those of a peri-menopausal woman. Your wife may experience vaginal dryness, pain with intercourse, lack of sex drive and night sweats or hot flashes. If she's not interested in having sex with you, cuddle instead. Show her you care without pressuring her for sex.

Your wife may be struggling with the big life questions like can she be a good mother? Is she up to the task? Don't compound potential feelings of inadequacy by acting disappointed and hurt if she doesn't want to have sex.

For most women, baby blues peak at two weeks post-partum, and then gradually subside. The best "instant cure" for a bout of the "weepys" is to get out of the house and go for a walk.

Your wife may not recognize if she's crossing the line between baby blues and post-partum depression. Post-partum depression is signified by feeling unable to take care of the baby, fear of holding or touching the baby, and possibly even thoughts of harming the baby or herself. You can recognize it before it gets dire if you witness increased frequency of crying jags, inability to get out of bed, lack of interest in self-care and hygiene, and expressions of anger or apathy at the baby.

If you're concerned your wife is experiencing post-partum depression talk to her about it. Don't hesitate to call her health care provider if you feel she doesn't recognize the depth of her depression, or if she's even in a depression. Left untreated, post-partum depression has serious consequences. Anti-depressants are very effective and usually only need to be taken for six to nine months for full recovery to transpire.

The Family Bed

The family bed is controversial. Some parents swear by it—bringing them closer to their spouse and child; others view it as a hindrance to their marriage and a way to "spoil" the child. It is definitely convenient. When the baby wants to nurse, mom can just roll to the side and nurse him without having to get out of bed.

You can't give a child too much love. If you prefer the family bed approach, go for it. Keep in mind though, that a child who sleeps with his parents can be very difficult to get out of the bed. This behavior can persist into early toddlerhood.

Dad's "Baby Blues": No Phase Lasts Forever

Did you know new dads are not immune to "baby blues"? The challenges of early parenthood differ from anything you've faced in the past and they can shake your confidence. A night of inconsolable crying can make you want to throw in the towel and crawl under a rock.

Discuss your feelings with your wife. Maybe you're both having the same feelings. You can work through anxiety together with breathing exercises, relaxation exercises, taking walks together and "talking it out". The mere act of "getting it off your chest" can lift both your spirits. Exercise such as walking together helps your body metabolize and rid itself of the toxins created by anxiety and negative feelings.

If these techniques don't work to counter your negative emotions and insecurities, engage in positive self talk. Use the "Socratic method" to balance each negative self statement with a positive one. For example, "I'll never survive this never-ending lack of sleep," can be turned into, "I will get through this difficult period one day at a time."

Above all rejoice in the opportunity your baby gives you for a new lease on life. It's the best chance you'll ever have at life's biggest "do-over". You can "fix" all the "mistakes" your parents made and give your child everything you wished you had while growing up. If you had a wonderful childhood, give that gift to your little one.

Office Notes: Matthew's story

"The big difference between having a baby at twenty-something and having a child at fifty is when you're in your twenties; it's more of just a getting through the day thing. You love your children but there are more intellectual challenges. You can easily get caught up in routine and monotony and lose sight of appreciation for the life you've brought into the world and how you have the ultimate power to impact that life.

At fifty you are more in touch with the feeling this child is a being created from love between two people. You're closer to the spiritual side of bringing a child into the world. You are more aware of your mortality and you understand your child is your legacy.

When I first held Ariana she was so small she took my breath away—there she was—and she wrapped her tiny fingers around mine; she could barely get them around my pinky because her fingers were so small.

When you make the choice to bring a child into the world, planned or not, you are responsible for that choice forever. Resolve to commit to his life fully.

The desire to procreate, have sex, is one of the strongest instincts. Understand the consequences of your choices to satisfy those instincts. If you're not ready to bring a child into the world, use birth control.

If you're a woman it's your body so you have the ultimate control and power over the choice. Don't rely on the man to do it because many men assume you've "taken care of it"—they still view it as your responsibility.

I see so many broken families out there and it doesn't have to be that way. By bringing a child into the world you've made a commitment to another human being—he didn't have any say in your choice, yet here he is—you and your desires, impulses, passion, all led to the moment of his creation.

So when you act, consider the ramifications of your behavior. Everything ripples out into the world. If you create a child and ignore that child you spread unhappiness in the world. On the other hand, if you nurture and honor her, your spirit shines as the sun. It rebounds and ricochets like diamonds of light glinting off the snow. In your child you become bound for all time to the future of the universe ..."

Epilogue

What I Learned From My Own Pregnancies and Births

I have two lovely children both of whom are growing up very fast.

Nothing really prepares you for pregnancy and birth other than going through it. My experiences awakened me to these processes in a way studying them and being an observer could not. I not only know what it's like to prescribe Terbutaline or bed rest for someone, I have experienced both.

I can discuss pain management for labor and epidurals from the perspective of someone who was determined to do "natural childbirth", then realized it really hurt too much to be worth being able to say "I did it naturally." Every woman's pain receptors are different and we each experience discomfort in a unique fashion. What's minimally painful for one woman may be excruciating for another.

I know what it's like to perform and to heal from a repair; and to have trouble with bladder leakage after birth. I understand what it's like to have difficulty getting a baby to latch on and manage other breast-feeding issues. I know what it's like to be up all night for several nights in a row with an inconsolable baby. I've both treated and experienced baby blues and post-partum depression.

I had preterm labor and was on bed rest with both pregnancies. During my son's pregnancy I was in my fourth year of residency and working one hundred hours per week with a lot of night call. I went into preterm labor at twenty-four weeks, was started on a Terbutaline pump, and placed on bed rest. I had to take a leave of absence until he was born; and make up the time at the end of my fourth year of residency. I probably could have prevented my preterm labor, had I cut back on my work hours. However, as a resident in obstetrics and gynecology at the time, I didn't have a choice. Ironically residents who took leaves of absence for medical reasons were looked upon as "weak" and treated with the respect of "lepers".

I returned to work at thirty-six weeks gestation and my son was born a week later at exactly thirty-seven weeks gestation. My water broke at one AM and he delivered at about one PM. I thought I would go "natural" without the epidural. That worked until I hit transition at seven centimeters. I was in the shower, managing my contractions with breathing and rocking, then all of a sudden I couldn't handle it. I needed something *now*. I sat down on the floor of the shower and my husband had to help me back to bed to get the epidural. When I received the epidural, I felt so much better and was able to enjoy my son's birth without having to just focus on managing the pain. His healthy, safe arrival amazed me and made it worth all the bedrest, Terbutaline, and missed work.

My son was delivered by an Obstetrician (M.D.) who I knew through my residency program. She was wonderful—supportive, non-paternalistic.

Four years later when I was pregnant with my daughter, I had moved to a different part of the state, and worked in a practice with two other physicians and two midwives. I wasn't working as many hours as I did as a resident, but I was still working sixty to eighty hours per week and doing night call.

I made it to twenty-eight weeks with my daughter before having preterm labor, and needing bed rest and Terbutaline … again. My ob care provider was a Certified Nurse Midwife (CNM), who was also my best friend.

My daughter delivered at exactly thirty-seven weeks gestation, just like my son. I washed the car late Sunday morning, went into labor and delivered at two PM. Labor was fast (two hours) and she was delivered by my best friend, the CNM. I probably could have delivered her at home but I knew from my first experience I definitely wanted the epidural. Forget the "natural" thing—labor hurts!

Stress and long work hours probably played a large factor in my having preterm labor with both pregnancies. I probably could have reduced my chances of preterm labor had I managed my stress level better and found some way to either adjust my work hours or cope better with the long hours and lack of sleep.

Both kids are doing great. They're smart and beautiful, despite the preterm labor and the long exposure to Terbutaline.

I had equally wonderful birth experiences with both my doctor for the first; and my midwife for the second.

At this point, the details of pregnancy and labor are somewhat fuzzy. What matters most now is my two perfect children.

About the Author

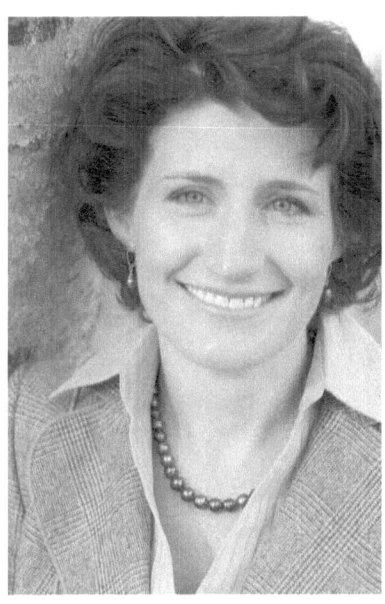

Dr. Binkley was born in Boulder, Colorado. She grew up all over the United States, but mostly in Philadelphia, PA. She has two beautiful smart children, and one beautiful smart husband. Dr. Binkley has practiced medicine in the Roaring Fork Valley of Colorado for the past twelve years and was awarded the 2006 "Local's Choice" Gold Award for "Best Ob-Gyn" by the Glenwood Springs Post Independent.

M.D. Temple University School of Medicine 1992
    Awarded "Best Student in Ob-Gyn" by Faculty and Residents
    Elected to Alpha Omega Alpha Honor Society
B.A. Swarthmore College 1988, "Distinction"
    Elected to Phi Beta Kappa Honor Society
Residency in Obstetrics and Gynecology at University of Colorado Health Sciences Center 1996

You can email the author at: info@alpinewomenscare.com

www.alpinewomenscare.com

www.drshelleybinkley.com

My Space page: myspace.com/shelleybinkley

Check out her blogs at blogspot.com/DIYBaby

References

Books

Cunningham, F. Gary, *et al. Williams Obstetrics, 21ˢᵗ Edition*. New York, New York: McGraw-Hill, 2001.

Gabbe, Steven G., et al. *Obstetrics: Normal and Problem Pregnancies*, Third Edition. New York, New York: Churchill Livingstone, 1996.

Articles on Home Birth

Bastian, Hilda, et al.1998. Perinatal death associated with planned home birth in Australia: population based study. *British Medical Journal* 317: 384–8.

Chamberlain, G. V. P. et al. 1998. What is really happening to home births? *Journal of Obstetrics and Gynecology* 18(1): 7–8.

Davies, J, et al. 1996. Prospective regional study of planned home births. British Medical Journal 313: 1302–6.

Durand, Mark A. 1992. The Safety of Home Birth: The Farm Study. *American Journal of Public Health* 82(3): 450–3.

Janssen, Patricia A. et al., 2002. Outcomes of planned home births versus planned hospital births after regulation of midwifery in British Colombia. *Canadian Medical Association Journal* 166(3): 315–thirty-two3.

Johnson, Kenneth C. and Daviss, Betty-Anne. 2005. Outcomes of planned home births with certified professional midwives: large prospective study in North America. *British Medical Journal* 330: 1416–1422.

Murphy, Patricia Aikins et al., 1998. Outcomes of Intended Home Births in Nurse Midwifery Practice: A Prospective Descriptive Study. *Obstet Gynecol* 92: 461–470.

Pang, Jenny W. Y. et al. 2002 Outcomes of Planned Home Births in Washington State: 1989–1996. *Obstet Gynecol* 100(2):253–9.

Remez, L. 1997. Planned home birth can be as safe as hospital delivery for women with low-risk pregnancies. *Family Planning Perspectives* 29(3): 141–3

Weigers, T A, et al. 1996. Outcome of planned home and planned hospital births in low risk pregnancies: prospective study in midwifery practices in the Netherlands. *British Medical Journal* 313: 1309–1313

Articles on General Pregnancy Topics
General

Hamilton, Brady E., et al. 2007 Births: Preliminary Data for 2006. *National Vital Statistics Reports*. 56(7): 1–21. (CDC Publication).

Operative Vaginal Delivery (Forceps and Vaccuum)

Caughey, Aaron B. et al. 2005. Forceps compared with vaccum. *Obstet Gynecol* 106(5): 908–912.

Preterm Labor and Preterm Birth

Ananth, Cande V. et al., 2005. Trends in preterm birth and perinatal mortality among singletons: United States, 1989 through 2000. *Obstet Gynecol* 105(5): 1084–91.

Gilbert, William M. et al. 1003 The cost of prematurity: Quantification by gestational age and birth weight. *Obstet Gynecol* 102(3): 488–92.

Screening Tests

Ewigman, Bernard G. et al for The RADIUS Study Group. 1993. Effect of prenatal ultrasound screening on perinatal outcome. *New England Journal of Medicine* thirty-two9: 821–7.

Malone, F et al for The FASTER Trial Group. 2005. First trimester or second trimester screening, or both, for Down's Syndrome. *New England Journal of Medicine* 353(19): 2001–2011.

Vaginal Birth After Cesarean

McMahon, Michael J. et al. 1999. Comparison of a trial of labor with an elective second cesarean section. *New England Journal of Medicine* 355(10): 689–695.

Index

Quick Order Form

Fax Orders: 970-945-4466. Send this form.

Telephone Orders: 970-945-4499. Have your credit card ready.

E-mail orders: books@alpinewomenscare.com.

Postal Order: Alpine Women's Care, Attn: Books, 1607 Grand Avenue, #31, Glenwood Springs, CO 81601

Please send the following books when they are available. I understand I may return any of them within thirty days for a full refund—for any reason, no questions asked.

☐ **Get A Grip! On Your Hormones**

☐ **Omit Needless Worry: Awakening Your Power to Manage Anxiety**

☐ **Let's Fix Health Care! 4 Easy Steps**

Name: _____

Address _____

City _____ State _____ Zip _____

E-mail address: _____

Telephone (for order inquiries): _____

Privacy Promise: This information will only be used to process your book order; and not be distributed in any form to a third party.

978-0-595-49851-2
0-595-49851-5

www.ingramcontent.com/pod-product-compliance
Lightning Source LLC
Chambersburg PA
CBHW030308290526
45785CB00001B/255